Praise for Jonathan Bailor Research and Program

"I am often asked when there will be a proven prescription for weight loss. This is that prescription."
- **Harvard Medical School's** Dr. Theodoros Kelesidis

"A treasure trove of reliable information...hot, hot hot!"
- **Harvard Medical School's** Dr. JoAnne Manson

"Reveals the real story of diet, exercise, and their effects on us. I heartily recommend this." - **Harvard Medical School's** Dr. John J. Ratey

"Opens the black box of fat loss and makes it simple!"
- **Dr. Oz's Personal Trainer** Joel Harper

"I'm a big fan" – **World's Top Trainer and Creator of P90X** Tony Horton

"Will do more to assist people with their health than all the diet books out there put together. I want to shout, 'Bravo! Finally someone gets it!'"
- Dr. Christiane Northrup, **New York Times best-selling author** of *Women's Bodies, Women's Wisdom* and *The Wisdom of Menopause*

"Provides a powerful set of tools for creating lifelong health!"
- Dr. Mark Hyman, **New York Times best-selling author** of *The Blood Sugar Solution* and *The Daniel Plan*

"An easily understood and applied framework that will change the way you live, look, and feel... will end your confusion once and for all."
- Dr. William Davis, **New York Times best-selling author** of *Wheat Belly*

"Cuts through the noise around weight loss and tells it to us straight."
- Dr. Sara Gottfried, **New York Times best-selling author** of *The Hormone Cure* and *The Hormone Reset Diet*

"Readers will find that focusing on the kinds of foods they are eating can boost their brain power and help them lose the extra ten pounds."
- Dr. Daniel G. Amen, **New York Times best-selling author** of *Change Your Brain, Change Your Body*

"Will change the way you look at dieting!"
- JJ Virgin, **New York Times best-selling author** of *The Virgin Diet*

See hundreds more medical reviews and success stories at:
www.SANESolution.com

To my best friend, partner, and wife, Angela. Just the thought of you brings me more joy, more satisfaction, and more life than anything else I have ever experienced. You are my beloved, without reservation or qualification, as we dance into eternity.

To my heroes and parents, Mary Rose and Robert. All that I am is thanks to your love, example, and support. From the day I was born, and every day after, you have always found a way to help and love me. I live, hoping to return the favor.

To my friends and partners, Scott, Tyler, Sean, Abhishek, April, Lori, Wednesday, Josh, Jason, Andrea, and Rebecca, my delightful sister Patty, my wonderful brothers Tim, Cameron, and Branden, and my loving in-laws Terry and Carolyn. You are such treasures. Thank you for being who you are and thank you for meaning so much to me.

To you and the hundreds of thousands of other SANE family members all around the world with the courage to eat and exercise smarter. You have taken the road less traveled and it will make all the difference.

Published in the Worldwide by Yopti, LLC (SANESolution) New York. Seattle. California. www.SANESolution.com.

SANE books can be purchased at quantity discounts to use as premiums, promotions, or for corporate training programs. For more information on bulk pricing please email Yopti, LLC at SANESolution.com/contact.

Editor: Mary Rose Bailor
Production: Abhishek Pandey
Exterior Design: Tyler Archer

Publisher's Cataloging-in-Publication
Bailor, Jonathan.
72 Calorie Myth and SANE Certified Dessert Recipes: Lose Weight, Increase Energy, Improve Your Mood, Fix Digestion, and Sleep Soundly With The Delicious New Science of SANE Eating/ Jonathan Bailor.—1st ed.
p. cm.
1. Health   2. Weight Loss   3. Cooking   4. Recipes   5. Diet   6. Nutrition
I. Bailor, Jonathan II. Title.

Manufactured in the United States of America. First Edition.

The information expressed here is intended for educational purposes only. This information is provided with the understanding that neither Jonathan Bailor nor Yopti, LLC nor SANESolution nor affiliates are rendering medical advice of any kind. This information is not intended to supersede or replace medical advice, nor to diagnose, prescribe or treat any disease, condition, illness or injury. It is critical before beginning any eating or exercise program, including those described in this and related works, that readers receive full medical clearance from a licensed physician.

Jonathan Bailor, Yopti, LLC, SANESolution, and affiliates are not liable to anyone or anything impacted negatively, or purported to have been impacted negatively, directly or indirectly, by leveraging this or related information. By continuing to read this and related works the reader accepts all liability and disclaims Jonathan Bailor, Yopti, LLC, SANESolution, and affiliates from any and all legal matters. If these terms are not acceptable, visit SANESolution.com/contact to return this for a full refund.

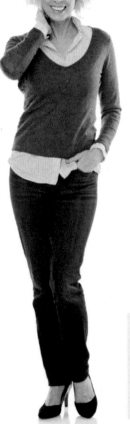

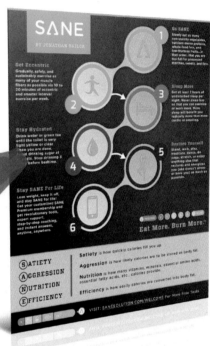
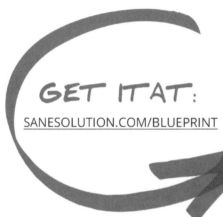
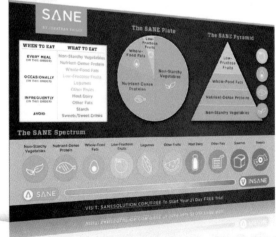
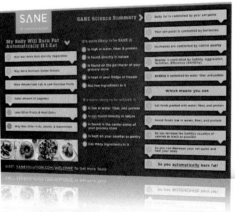

TABLE OF CONTENTS

TIP: Not familiar with the SANE Food Group or SANE Serving Sizes?

It's all good! Get everything you need by attending your FREE masterclass at SANESeminar.com and by downloading your FREE tools at SANESolution.com/Tools.

INTRODUCTION

Welcome to the SANE family! Jonathan Bailor here and I want to thank you again for taking time out of your hectic schedule to ensure that **your dinner table is for savoring and smiles, not self-criticism and calorie math**. Eating should be a source of joy and wellness, not shame and sickness. I sincerely hope that our time together will open your eyes to how easy it can be to reach your weight and fitness goals once you break free from the confusing and conflicting outdated theories and lies that have trapped you for so long.

If you only take one thing away from this book let it be this: **Any weight problem you may be experiencing is not your fault!** I know that may sound trite, but it's true. How can you be expected to lose those annoying pounds when all you've been given is outdated science and methods from the 1960's that have been proven NOT to work.

My mission is to not only reshape your body, but it's also to reshape the way you think about weight loss. What that means is I will be here with you every step of the way to provide all the support and tools you need to finally reach your weight loss goals. Whether you need to lose a few extra pounds around your belly, are looking for a **complete body transformation,** want **all-day energy,** or just want to make sense of all the confusing and conflicting health information out there once and for all, you are **finally in the right place!**

TIP: Be sure to add service@SANESolution.com to your email safe senders list/address book. This ensures you get all your upcoming SANE bonus recipes, tools, and how-to videos.

So if you are ready to stop counting calories... Ready to stop killing yourself with exercise you hate... Ready to end your struggle with weight... and are tired of being hungry and tired...this is your chance. It's time to get off the dieting roller-coaster once and for all. **Are you ready?**

I urge you to make a commitment to yourself to continue this journey. You are worth it. After all, you took action to get this book so that means you are ready and willing to step up and make positive changes. If you follow the simple and scientifically backed principles we teach, **I promise you will lose weight...and keep it off for good.**

You are part of the family now, and I am so excited to have you here as we bust the myths that have been holding you back... perhaps for years. Remember this...**now is your time**, and these are your proven tools for lasting weight loss success. Welcome home.

Can't wait to meet you at SANESolution.com,

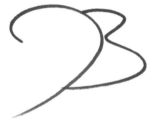

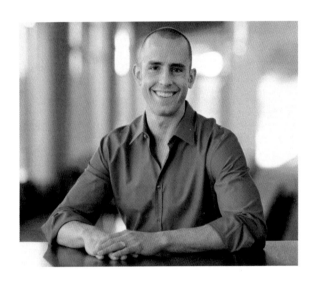

Jonathan Bailor
New York Times Bestselling Author,
SANE Founder, and soon...your
personal weight-loss coach

P.S. Over the years I have found that our most successful members, the ones who have lost 60, 70, even 100 pounds...and kept it off...are the ones who started their personal weight-loss plan on our FREE half-day Masterclass. It's your best opportunity to fall in love with the SANE lifestyle, learn exactly how to start making the simple changes that lead to dramatic body transformations, and get introduced to your new SANE family. **Be sure to reserve your spot now at http://SANESeminar.com.**

ENDLESS VARIETY AND SANE SUBSTITUTION (VS. DEPRIVATION)

Going SANE isn't about deprivation. It's about enjoying so much good food that you are too full for the sickening stuff. Even better, there are A LOT of delicious recipes that do not require unnatural, fattening, toxic, and addictive ingredients :) In fact, chocolate is the most craved food in the world, and the ingredient that puts the "c" in chocolate—cocoa—is spectacularly SANE.

Keeping "substitution rather than deprivation" principle in mind, you can cook and eat almost anything by making some simple swaps. While these swaps will taste slightly different, they will also make you look and feel completely different—a tradeoff that you will very much enjoy long term. The following cheat sheet will get you started SANEly swapping your way to slimness.

The best thing about this SANE swap approach is that it means that you have access to an endless supply of SANE recipes. All you need to do is find a recipe you like, and then SANEitize it! For example, some of the *SANECertified*™ recipes here were inspired by amazing semi-SANE recipes found around the web. Be sure to check out an ever-growing list of our favorite sites for SANEitizable recipe inspiration at http://bit.ly/InspireSANESubstitution.

> *Inspiration + SANE Substitutions = Endless Variety = :)*

If you would like help with making SANE substitutions, please attend our free interactive masterclass webinar at http://SANESeminar.com.

SANE Substitution Cheat Sheet

inSANE	SANE
Pasta & Rice	• Spaghetti squash/Squoodles • Zucchini noodles/Zoodles • Shirataki noodles • Shredded cabbage • Shaved brussels sprouts • Bean sprouts • Pea shoots • Cauliflower rice • Broccoli and carrot slaw (premade in grocery produce section)
Potatoes	• Mashed cauliflower • Turnips • Eggplant • Squash • Zucchini
Bread, Cookies, Cakes, Pies, Waffles, Pancakes, and Tortillas	• Baked goods made using golden flaxseed meal, coconut flour, almond meal, almond flour, and other nut flours • Low-carb and diabetic breads, tortillas, etc. that contain as few ingredients as possible • Clean Whey Protein • SANE Bars & Energy Bites
Hot and cold cereal	• SANE cereals made with coconut flour, chia, ground flax, and nuts.
Pretzels & chips	• SANE Bake-N-Crisps • Nuts • Seeds • Baked kale chips
Candy Bars, Energy Bars & Drinks, Chocolate	• SANE Bars & Energy Bites

TIP: Not familiar with the SANE Food Group or SANE Serving Sizes?

It's all good! Get everything you need by attending your FREE masterclass at **SANESeminar.com** and by downloading your FREE tools at **SANESolution.com/Tools**.

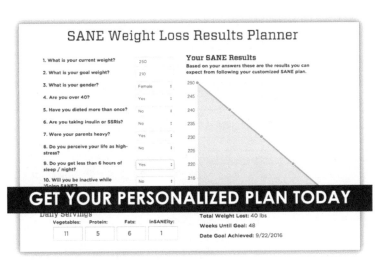
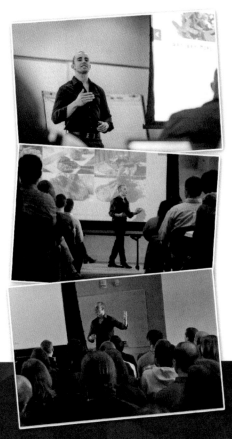

ALL PURPOSE SANE BAKING MIX

Total Time: 5 min
Prep: 5 min
Cook: 0 min

12 Servings
1 Whole-Food Fat Per Serving

Ingredients

- 1 cup Chia Seeds (or flax seeds)
- 1 cup Psyllium Husk
- 1 cup Coconut Flour
- 1 cup Unflavored Gelatin

- 1 cup Clean Whey Protein (only unflavored whey will work as you don't want this to add flavor)
- 2 TBSP Baking Powder
- 1/2 TSP Salt
- 1 TBSP Guar Gum (optional)

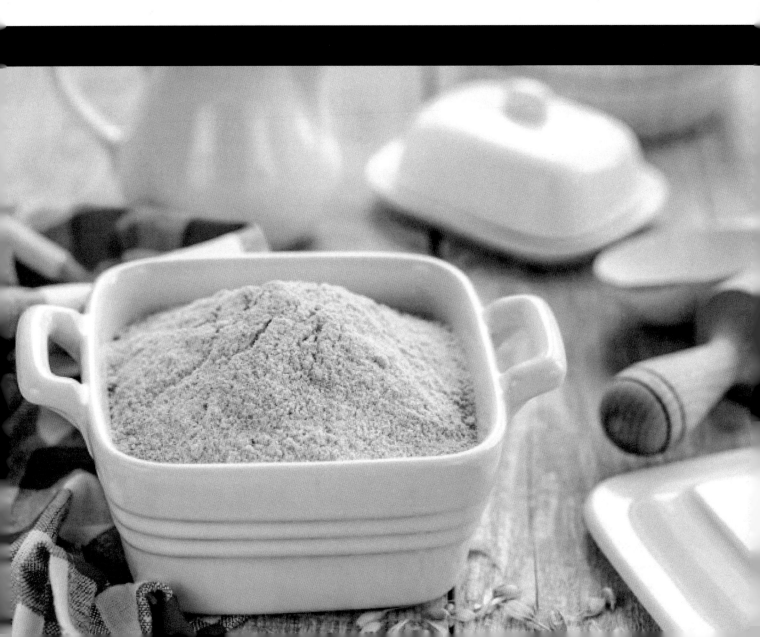

Directions

1. Combine all ingredients in a large bowl and mix thoroughly.

2. Place one or two cups at a time into a food processor or blender and pulverize completely into a fine flour-like powder.

3. IMPORTANT: The flax or chia seeds must be completely pulverized into a flour-like consistency. If your food processor or blender does not do this, please use flax meal as it is pre-pulverized.

4. Tip: Completely pulverized means you do not see "bits" of anything in the mixture. It is one homogeneous flour.

5. Once completely pulverized, remove from the food processor or blender.

6. Repeat steps 2 & 3 for the entire batch.

TIP: One serving is a rounded 1/3 cup

TIP: Ideal options for flax, chia, coconut flour, and clean whey can be found in your SANEStore by clicking here. Guar gum is optional and can be found on Amazon here.

TIP: If you use chia instead of flax (recommended), you may need to adjust the amount of water used with this flour as chia reacts much differently with liquid than flax.

APPLE CRISP

Total Time: 40min
Prep: 5 min
Cook: 35 min

8 Servings
1 Whole-Food Fat Per Serving
1 Other Fruits

Ingredients

- 2 lbs of apples
- 1/2 cup Coconut Flour
- 1/2 cup Almond Flour
- 1/2 cup gluten free oats
- 2/3 cup Xylitol
- 1/2 tsp Cinnamon
- 1/2 tsp Nutmeg

- 1/2 tsp All spice
- 1/4 tsp Sea salt
- 1/3 cup Extra Virgin Coconut Oil
- 2 tbsp Flax seed
- 2 tbsp Egg whites
- 1 tsp Vanilla

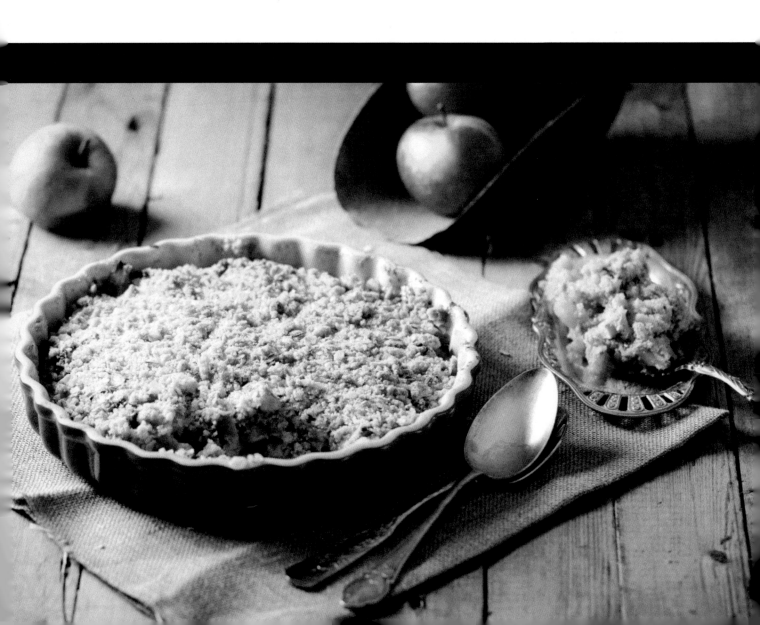

Directions

1. Preheat oven to 375

2. Core and slice apples.

3. Toss apples with a light sprinkle of cinnamon before placing in 8×11 (inch) glass dish

4. Separately, mix the egg whites and the flax seed together and let sit until needed

5. Add all remaining dry ingredients together in a bowl and mix up with a fork

6. Next add melted extra virgin coconut oil and vanilla along with the egg white & flax mixture

7. Mix together with fork until it creates a nice crumble

8. Spread evenly across the apples in the dish until completely covered

9. Bake for 30 minutes.

10. Once finished, let cool for at least another 30 minutes or so.

BITTERSWEET BROWNIE DROPS

Total Time: 25 min
Prep: 15 min
Cook: 10 min

12 Servings
1 Whole-Food Fat Per Serving

Ingredients

- 4 tbsps Almond Flour
- 1/2 tsp Baking Powder
- 3 ozs Unsweetened Baking Chocolate Squares
- 2 tbsps Unsalted Butter

- 1/2 - 3/4 cup Xylitol (adjust for personal sweetness)
- 2 large Eggs (Whole)
- 1/2 tsp Coconut Flour
- 1/4 tsp Vanilla Extract
- 1/4 tsp Baking Soda

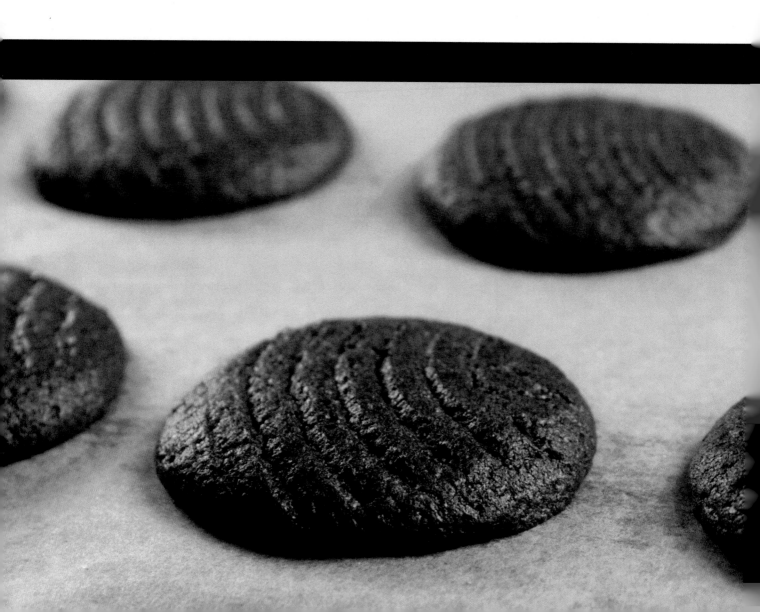

Directions

1. Preheat oven to 375°F. Line a baking sheet with parchment paper lightly greased with coconut oil or aluminum foil.

2. In a small bowl whisk almond flour, baking powder, baking soda and coconut flour.

3. In a microwave-safe bowl, melt chocolate and butter for 1 to 2 minutes, until butter is melted and chocolate has softened. (You can also do this step on the stovetop.)

4. Let stand 2 minutes and vanilla and stir until smooth.

5. With an electric mixer on medium speed, beat eggs and sugar substitute until light and fluffy, about 3 minutes.

6. Gradually beat the slightly warm chocolate mixture into the egg mixture until well-blended, about 1 minute.

7. Turn mixer speed down to low and mix in flour mixture just combined.

8. Drop slightly rounded teaspoonfuls of dough onto prepared sheet. Bake 5 to 6 minutes, until just set but still soft on top.

9. Gently remove pan from oven, let cookies cool for 5 minutes on pan (****very important or cookies will go super flat as they deflate when moved too early...think soufflé)

10. Transfer to a wire rack to cool completely.

BLACK VELVET CUPCAKES

Total Time: 22 min
Prep: 5 min
Cook: 17 min

6 Servings
2 Whole-Food Fats Per Serving

Ingredients

- 3 large Eggs (Whole)
- 1/4 cup Coconut Milk Unsweetened
- 1/3 cup Xylitol
- 2 tsps Vanilla Extract
- 7 tbsps Unsalted Butter

- 1/4 cup Almond Flour
- 1/4 tsp Baking Powder
- 2 tbsps SANE Cocoa Powder
- 1/4 tsp Baking Soda
- 1/4 tsp Salt
- 4 ozs Coconut Cream

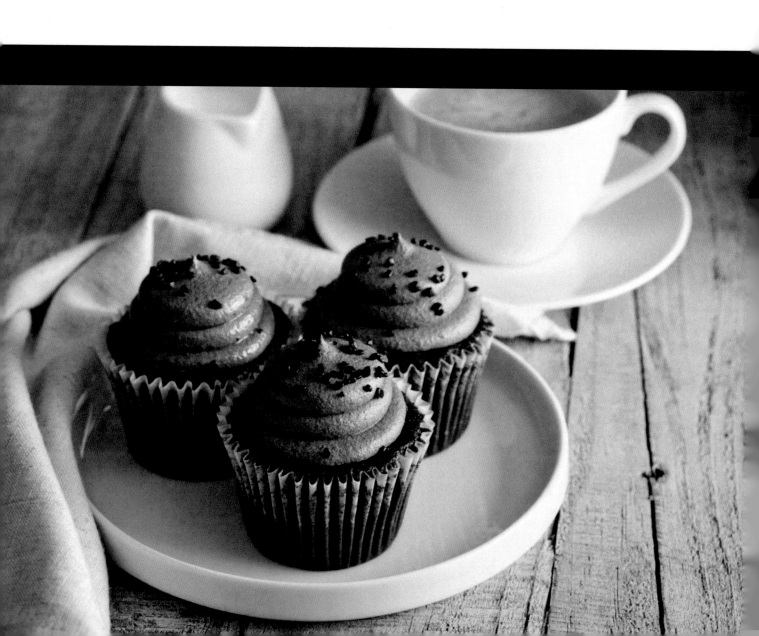

Directions

1. Preheat oven to 375°F. Prepare a muffin tin with 6 paper cups. Set aside.

2. In a medium bowl whisk the eggs with the coconut milk, 1/4 cup xylitol, vanilla, black food coloring and 3 tablespoons melted butter. Set aside.

3. In a small bowl whisk together the almond flour, baking powder, SANE Cocoa Powder, baking soda and salt. Add to egg mixture whisking to incorporate all ingredients for about a minute. Divide batter into the 6 paper cups, place in the oven and bake until fully set in the center; about 15-18 minutes. When done, set on a wire rack to cool.

4. Make Frosting: In a small bowl, beat the coconut cream with an electric mixer until smooth. Add 4 tbsp (1/4 cup) softened butter and continue to beat another minute. Add the remaining xylitol; beat another minute then add vanilla and food coloring as desired. Adjust for sweetness by adding a pinch of stevia if desired. Frost cupcakes using a piping bag or by hand.

BLUEBERRY CHEESECAKE TARTLETS

Total Time: 6hr 40 min
Prep: 20 min
Cook: 40 min

12 Servings
1 Whole-Food Fat Per Serving

Ingredients

- 2 cups Almond Flour
- 2 ozs SANE Cocoa Powder
- 10 tbsp Xylitol
- 1/4 cup Unsalted Butter
- 6 ozs Coconut Cream

- 1/2 cup Ricotta Cheese (Whole Milk)
- 2 large Eggs (Whole)
- 1/2 tsp Vanilla Extract
- 1 cup Fresh Blueberries
- 1 tbsp Tap Water
- 1 large Egg Yolk

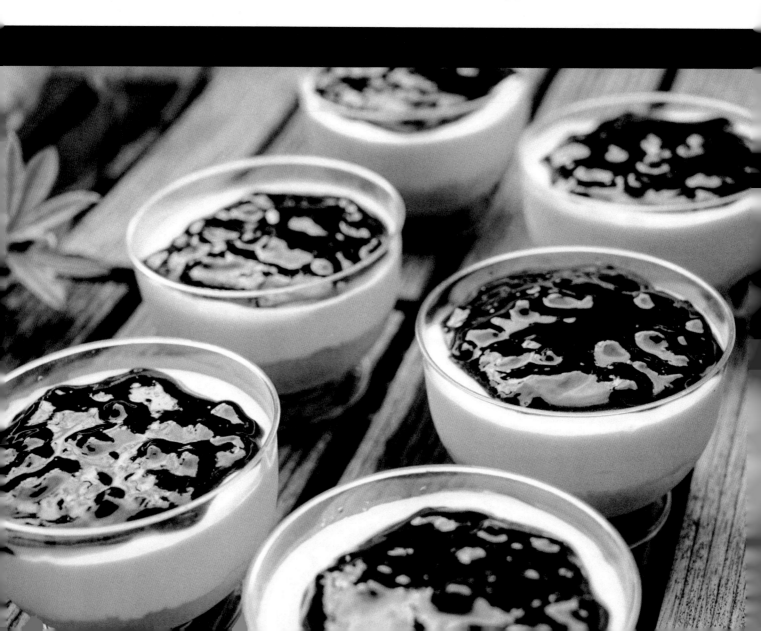

Directions

1. Preheat oven to 350°F. Liberally grease the cups of a 12-cup muffin tin, or 2 x 12 mini muffin pans or use muffin papers. In a medium bowl, whisk together almond meal, 3 tablespoons SANE Cocoa Powder, and Xylitol.

2. Pour in butter and stir with fork until it forms coarse crumbs. Place one heaping tablespoon of almond crust into the bottom of each mini muffin tin or about 2 1/2 tablespoons in the regular muffin tin wells or paper cups.

3. Using your fingers, press gently to work dough down and up the sides of the tin. Repeat until all muffin tins are filled. Place pan in oven and bake 5-7 minutes. Remove from oven and let cool.

4. Place coconut cream, ricotta cheese, eggs, vanilla, 1 tablespoon SANE Cocoa Powder, and Xylitol into a blender, and puree until smooth and free of lumps.

5. Pour coconut cream mixture evenly into cooled crusts, leaving 1/4-inch rim of space at the top of each cup.

6. Place pan back in oven and bake for 30-35 minutes for large muffin tins or 10-12 minutes for mini muffin tins, until the batter is no longer wet and firms around the edges. Remove from heat and let cool to room temperature.

7. Prepare the topping. In a small saucepan, add blueberries and water over medium heat. Bring to simmer, mashing blueberries with the back of a wooden spoon, until blueberries are hot and have released their juices.

8. Place your egg yolk in a small bowl. Whisking swiftly and continuously, add a tablespoon of warm blueberry juice to yolks to temper. Repeat again two more times until yolk is tempered.

9. Whisking quickly and constantly, pour tempered yolk into pan with blueberries. Stir, cooking, until blueberries are significantly thickened. Remove from heat and let cool slightly. Set aside to cool.

10. Spoon blueberry topping evenly over the tops of the cheesecake cups, spreading to cover evenly. Place muffin tin in refrigerator and let cool 4-5 hours or overnight, until chilled completely. To serve, carefully pop cheesecake cups out of muffin tin and place on serving tray. Two per person if using the mini muffin tins or 1 per person if using the regular muffin tins.

BLUEBERRY COBBLER

Total Time: 1hr 10 min
Prep: 10 min
Cook: 1hr

12 Servings
1 Whole-Food Fat Per Serving

Ingredients

- 3 cups washed blueberries
- 2 cups almond flour
- 1/4 cup coconut flour
- 1/2 tsp baking soda
- 1/4 tsp sea salt
- 1/2 cup SANE honey

- 1/4 cup butter, soft
- Drop of almond extract
- 3 tbsp flax-meal whisked with 9 tbsp warm water, allowed to plump up for 5 minutes
- 1 tbsp apple cider vinegar (to be added last)

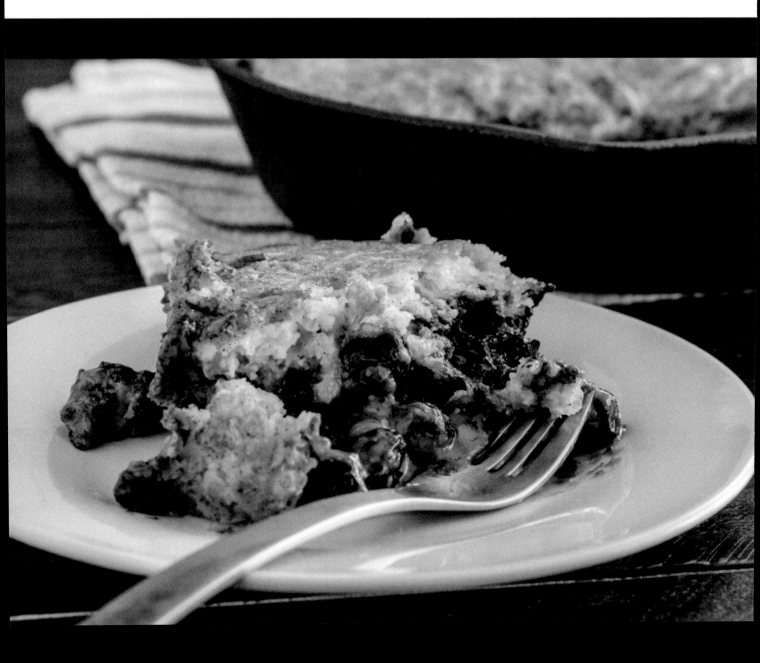

Directions

1. Preheat oven to 350 degrees F.

2. Grease an 8×8 glass dish with extra virgin coconut oil.

3. Pour the Blueberries in pan, reserving a few berries for the top if you wish.

4. Whisk the almond flour, salt, and baking soda in a bowl.

5. Separately, whisk together butter, honey, and extract.

6. Mix wet and dry ingredients together, stirring in the flax. Once well combined, quickly stir in cider vinegar.

7. Pour batter onto berries, spreading up to the edges.

8. Bake for 40 minutes, or until batter is set on top. this happens to vary in my house, sometimes taking 50 minutes.

CARAMEL CHOCOLATE BROWNIES

Total Time: 35 min
Prep: 5 min
Cook: 30 min

9 Servings
1 Whole-Food Fat Per Serving

Ingredients

- 1/4 cup coconut flour
- 1 1/4 cup SANE Cocoa Powder
- 4 eggs
- 1 tsp sea salt
- 1 tsp baking soda
- 1/2 cup SANE honey

- 1/4 cup Xylitol
- 1 tbsp vanilla extract
- 1/3 cup extra virgin coconut oil
- 1/3 cup dark chocolate chips
- 1 homemade caramel recipe

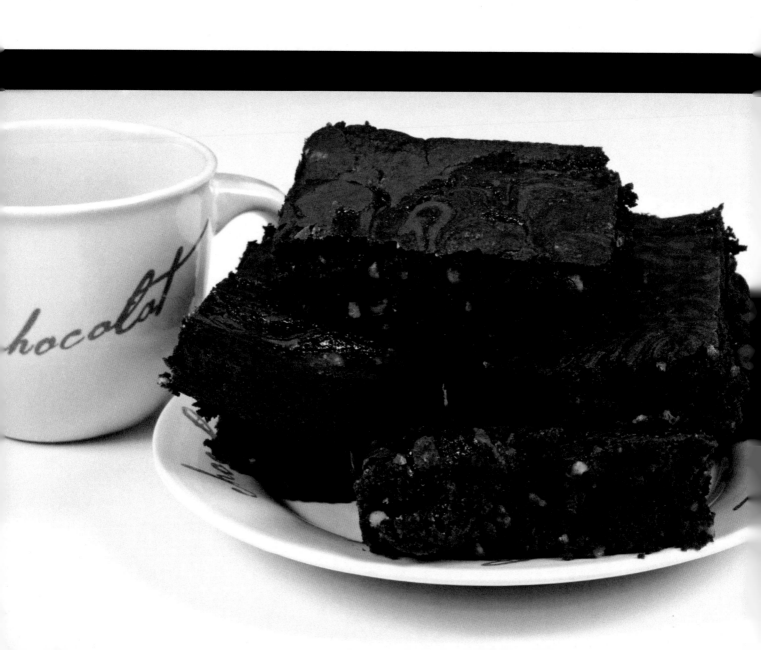

Directions

1. Preheat oven to 350 degrees Fahrenheit.

2. Mix dry ingredients in one bowl and wet ingredients in a second bowl.

3. Combine both mixtures and stir until all ingredients are incorporated together.

4. Pour the mixture into a greased 8×8 pan.

5. Top with chocolate chips and/or nuts if desired, and bake for 25-30 minutes.

6. Let cool and then drizzle with caramel sauce.

CARAMELIZED PEAR CUSTARD

Total Time: 30 min
Prep: 10 min
Cook: 20 min

8 Servings
2 Whole-Food Fats Per Serving

Ingredients

- 2 tbsps Butter
- 2 tbsps Xylitol
- 1/4 tsp ground Cardamom
- 2 medium Pears
- 3 large Eggs (Whole)

- 2 large Egg Yolks
- 2 cups Coconut Cream
- 1/8 cup Sugar Free Maple Flavor Syrup
- 1/2 fl oz Rum
- 1 tsp Vanilla Extract

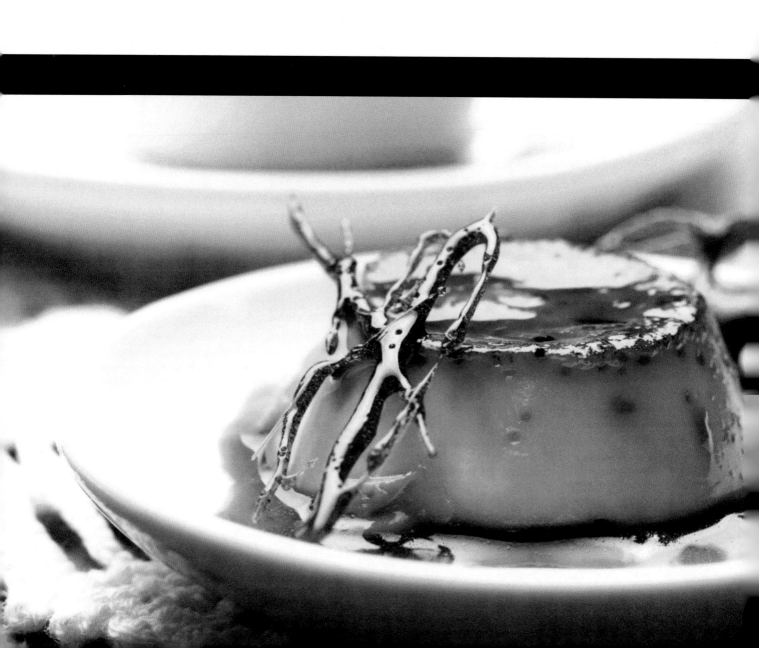

Directions

1. Preheat oven to 375°F.

2. Heat the butter, xylitol and cardamom in a large sauce pan over medium-high heat. Slice the pears into 1/2-inch wedges. Once the butter has melted add the pears and allow to caramelized for 4 minutes on each side. Remove from heat and arrange in a pie plate or 3-4 cup casserole dish. Reserve about 2 Tbsp purée of xylitol and pour the remaining over the pears (keep remaining in the sauce pan and set aside).

3. In a small bowl, whisk the eggs, egg yolks, coconut cream, purée of xylitol, rum and vanilla until combined. Pour mixture over the pears and bake for 15-20 minutes until golden brown and custard has set. Remove from oven and allow to cool slightly.

4. Using a pastry brush, brush the top with reserved a purée of xylitol.

Chocolate Chip-Macadamia Nut
Ice Cream Sandwiches

Total Time: 6hr 25 min   10 Servings
Prep: 6hr   3 Whole-Food Fats Per Serving
Cook: 25 min

Ingredients

- 3 cups Coconut Cream
- 3 tbsps Unsalted Butter
- 1/2 cup whole or halved Macadamia Nuts
- 3 large Egg Yolks

- 1 tbsp Tap Water
- 1/4 tsp Salt
- 2 tsps Vanilla Extract
- 3/4 cup Xylitol
- 1/2 tsp Pure Almond Extract
- 3 large Eggs (Whole)

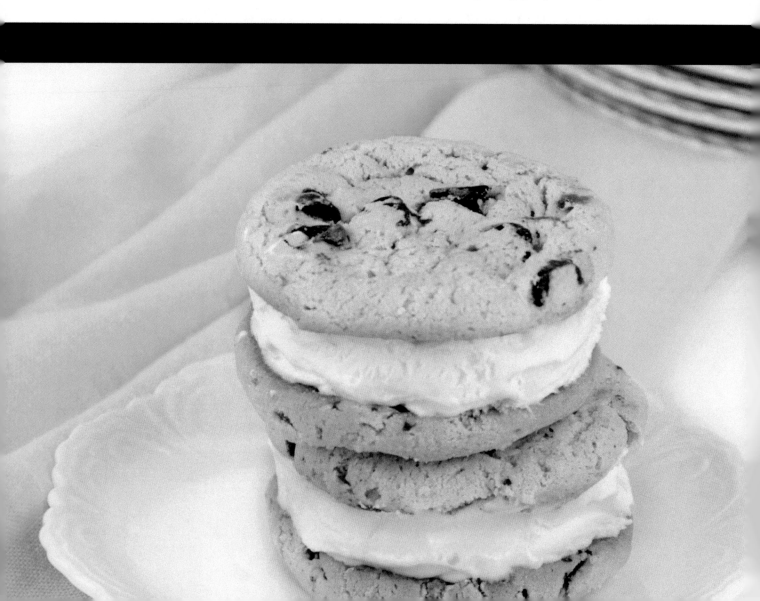

Directions

1. For the cookies: Mix according to package directions, adding the butter, 1 egg and water. Portion the dough to make 20 cookies. Bake and cool following the package directions; set aside.

2. For the macadamia nut ice cream: Pour coconut cream into a heavy-bottomed 3-quart saucepan and place over medium heat. Bring to a low boil, stirring often so the cream does not boil over. Remove from heat. In a large bowl, place 2 eggs, egg yolks, xylitol and salt. Using either a hand mixer or a whisk, beat together until thickened and smooth.

3. Using a ladle, remove about a cup of the hot cream from saucepan and gradually whisk into egg mixture. Whisking, pour tempered egg mixture into remaining cream in saucepan.

4. Place over medium heat and whisk until slightly thickened, 1 to 2 minutes. Pour into a clean bowl, whisk in vanilla and almond extracts; let stand until custard is completely cooled to room temperature, about 1 ½ hours.

5. Refrigerate 2 hours, until well chilled, or cover with plastic wrap and refrigerate overnight. Freeze in ice cream maker according to manufacturers directions. Add chopped macadamia nuts 15 minutes before freezing process is complete.

6. To assemble sandwiches: Arrange 10 cookies, top side down, on work surface. Using an ice cream scoop, working quickly, place 1/4 cup ice cream on each cookie. Top each with another cookie, bottom side down.

7. Wrap each sandwich well in plastic wrap and place in freezer. Freeze at least 4 hours (ice cream will be soft) or overnight (for firmer sandwiches). Can be stored in the freezer up to 1 month.

Chocolate Chunk Bars

Total Time: 30 min
Prep: 10 min
Cook: 20 min

16 Servings
1 Whole-Food Fat Per Serving

Ingredients

- 1/4 cup Melted Extra Virgin Coconut Oil
- 1/3 cup SANE honey
- 2 teaspoons Vanilla Extract
- 2 eggs, Slightly Beaten
- 1/4 cup Unsweetened almond milk

- 1/2 cup Coconut Flour
- 1/2 teaspoon Baking soda
- 1/4 teaspoon Salt
- 3 oz Dark chocolate bar, coarsely chopped
- 1/2 cup coconut flakes, optional

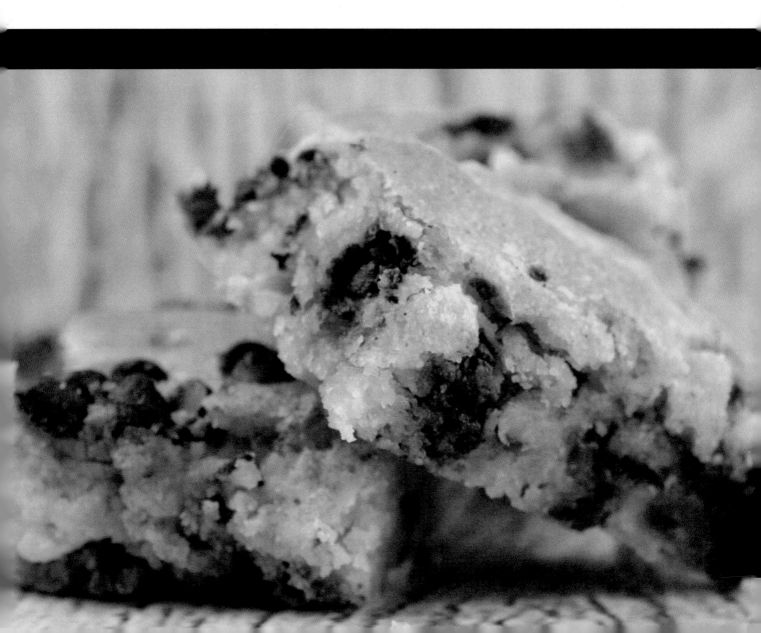

Directions

1. Preheat oven to 350 degrees F. Spray 8×8 inch baking pan with nonstick cooking spray.

2. In a large bowl, whisk together extra virgin coconut oil, SANE honey, vanilla, eggs, and almond milk. In a separate medium bowl whisk together coconut flour, baking soda, and salt. Add dry ingredients to wet ingredients and mix until just combined and batter is smooth. Fold in chopped chocolate, reserved a few tablespoons for sprinkling on top if desired.

3. Bake for 20-22 minutes or until edges are golden brown and knife comes out with a few crumbs attached. The batter may look like it's not all the way cooked but it will be. DO NOT OVERBAKE or it will result in dried out bars and no one likes that! I always bake mine for 20 minutes and don't have any problems. Cool bars on a wire rack for at least 10 minutes so that they settle a bit, then cut into 16 squares. Enjoy!

Mini Chocolate Cups

Total Time: 20 min
Prep: 20 min
Cook: 0 min

1 Serving
1 Whole-Food Fat Per Serving

Ingredients

- 1 1/2 ozs Sugar Free Chocolate Chips

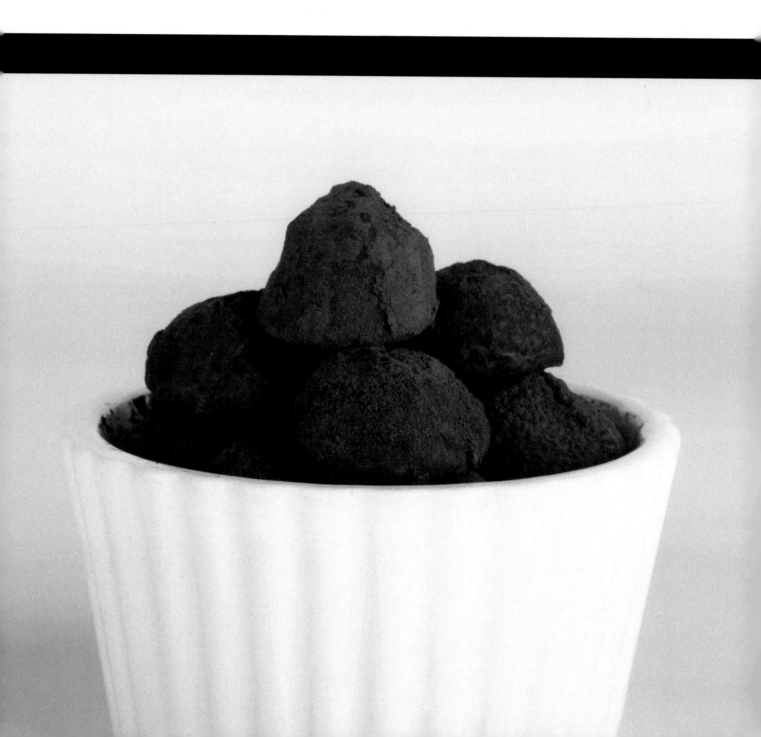

Directions

1. Line a mini muffin tin compartment with a paper cupcake liner. Place chocolate pieces in a Pyrex measuring cup. Microwave on 20 percent power for 30 seconds. Stir, and repeat process until pieces are melted but haven't completely lost their shape. Stir until smooth.

2. With a pastry brush, coat inside of cupcake liner with a layer of chocolate. Refrigerate 4 to 5 minutes, until chocolate sets. Repeat process until all the chocolate is used up. When chocolate is hardened, carefully peel off liner.

3. Cups may be made ahead, covered in plastic and stored in a cool place for up to 5 days.

Chocolate Donuts

Total Time: 18 min
Prep: 5 min
Cook: 13 min

6 Servings
1 Whole-Food Fat Per Serving

Ingredients

- 1 large Egg (Whole)
- 4 ozs Almond Butter
- 2 tbsps SANE Cocoa Powder
- 2 tbsps Erythritol

- 1/4 tsp Baking Powder
- 1/4 tsp Baking Soda
- 1/4 tsp Salt
- 7 oz Coconut Cream
- 2 tsps Vanilla Extract

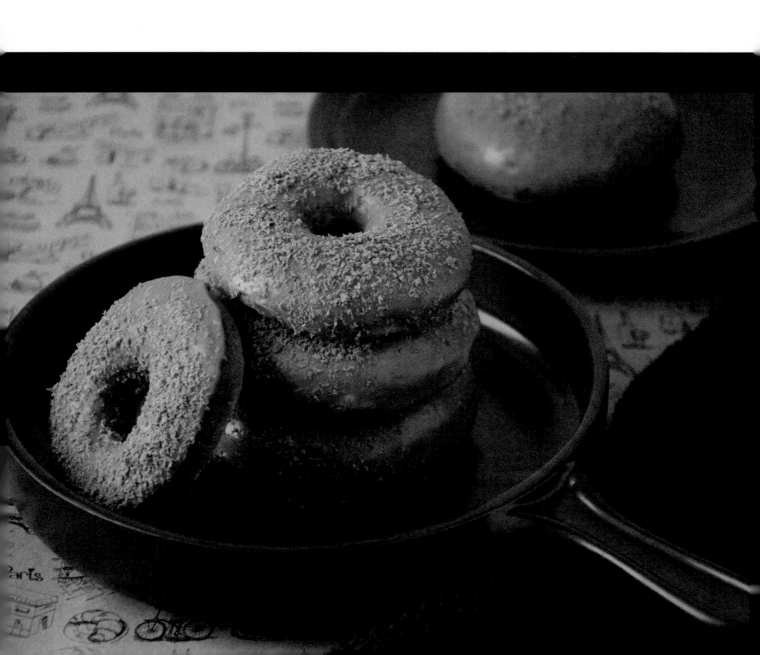

Directions

1. Preheat oven to 350°F. Prepare a 6-well donut pan with non-stick spray.

2. Place all ingredients in a blender or food processor, pulse a few times, scraping the container between pulses.

3. Pour into donut pan and bake for 13 minutes. Cool in pan for 10 minutes then turn out on a wire rack to cool completely.

Chocolate Ganache Macarons

Total Time: 55 min
Prep: 15 min
Cook: 40 min

20 Servings
1 Whole-Food Fat Per Serving

Ingredients

- 3 large Egg Whites
- 1 tsp Fresh Lemon Juice
- 1/4 cup cocoa powder

- 1/2 cup Almond Flour
- 4 tbsps Xylitol
- 6 ozs 100% cocoa baking chocolate
- 2 tbsps Coconut Cream

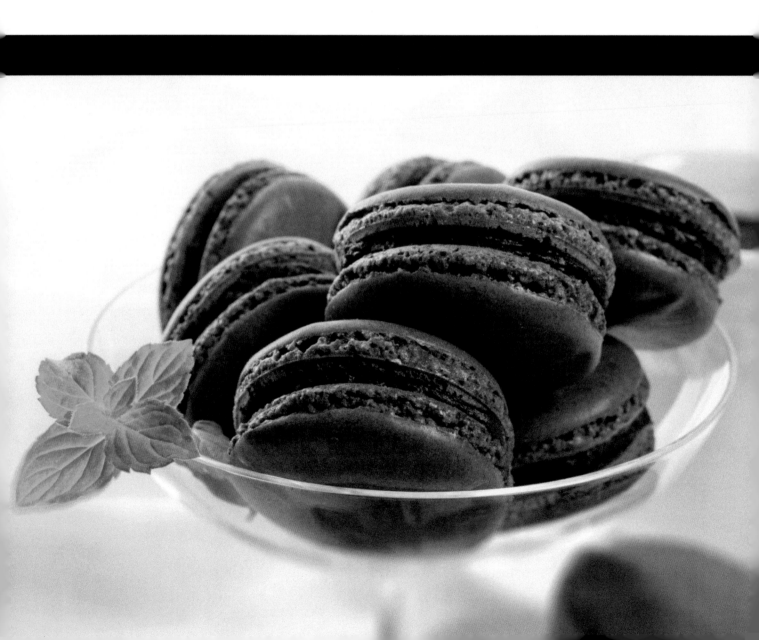

Directions

1. Preheat oven to 250°F. Prepare a silicon baking mat or parchment paper on a baking sheet. Drawing 1-inch circles on the backside of the parchment can be helpful. Set aside.

2. Using a stand mixer with the whip attachment, whip the egg whites, lemon juice, a pinch of salt and 1 tablespoon of the xylitol until stiff peaks form.

3. Sift together 1 tablespoon xylitol, almond flour, and cocoa powder.

4. Add to the egg whites and gently fold in to fully incorporate.

5. Using a piping bag or simply cut the end of a large zippered plastic bag, fill with the meringue and pipe onto the baking sheet making 1-inch rounds.

6. Tap the tops with a slightly wet finger if tips remain. Bake for 35-45 minutes. If they begin to brown, decrease temperature by 25 degrees and bake a little longer. Remove from oven and allow to cool down. Once cooled remove with a spatula and set on a fresh piece of parchment paper.

7. Make Filling: melt chocolate in the microwave at 30 second intervals.

8. Add coconut cream and remaining 2 tbsp of xylitol using a handheld blender; whip until thick.

9. Using a small piping bag, pipe chocolate onto the flat side of 1 macaron then top with the another on the flat side sandwiching together.

10. Sprinkle with a little cocoa powder as a garnish if desired

Chocolate Mousse Mini Cheesecakes

Total Time: 5hr
Prep: 4hr 30 min
Cook: 30 min

8 Servings
3 Whole-Food Fats Per Serving

Ingredients

- 3 ozs Unsweetened Baking Chocolate Squares
- 3 cup Coconut Cream
- 1/2 cup Xylitol
- 3 large Eggs (Whole)
- 3/4 tsp Pure Almond Extract
- 1/2 tsp Vanilla Extract

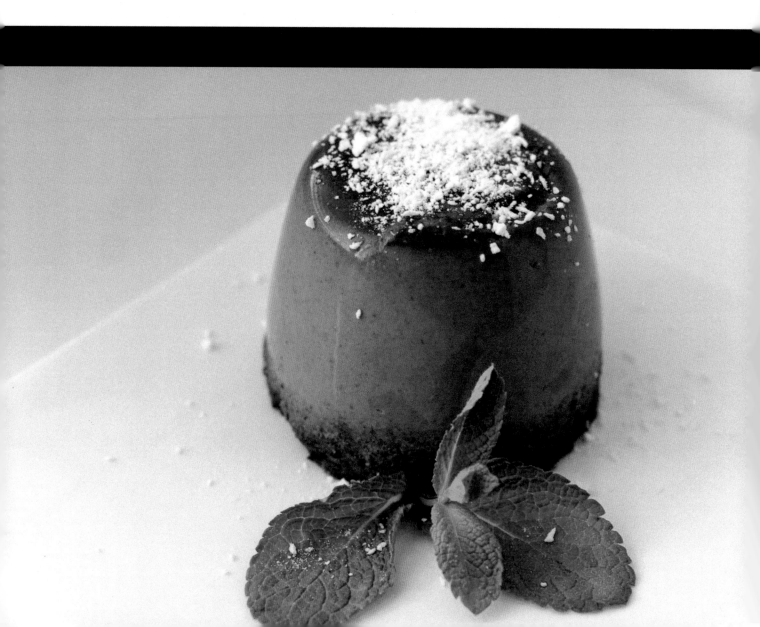

Directions

1. Heat oven to 325°F.

2. Place eight 6-ounce ramekins in a roasting pan; set aside.

3. Heat chocolate in the microwave in 30-second increments until fully melted, about 1-2 minutes; set aside to cool slightly.

4. In the large bowl of an electric mixer, beat 2 cup coconut cream on medium speed until lightened, scraping down sides of bowl as needed. Add chocolate and beat until combined. Add xylitol, beating until combined.

5. Add eggs, one at a time, beating well after each addition. Add one cup coconut cream and almond and vanilla extracts, beating until completely smooth.

6. Pour mixture into prepared custard cups. Carefully pour enough boiling water into roasting pan to come halfway up sides of ramekins.

7. Bake until the cheesecakes are puffed and the centers are just set, about 20 minutes. Remove from oven and let sit in the water bath for 10 minutes.

8. Transfer custard cups to a wire rack; cool to room temperature. Refrigerate until well chilled, 4 hours or overnight.

9. Garnish with mint sprigs, chocolate shavings and raspberries, if desired.

Chocolate Peppermint Cupcakes

Total Time: 32 min
Prep: 15 min
Cook: 17 min

6 Servings
2 Whole-Food Fats Per Serving

Ingredients

- 3 large Eggs (Whole)
- 1/4 cup Coconut Milk Unsweetened
- 1/4 cup Xylitol
- 1 tsp Vanilla Extract
- 7 tbsps Unsalted Butter
- 4 tbsps Almond Flour

- 2 tbsps SANE Cocoa Powder
- 1/4 tsp Baking Powder
- 1/4 tsp Salt
- 4 ozs Coconut Cream
- 2 tbsps Erythritol
- 1 serving Bob's Starlight Mints Peppermint Sugar Free Candy

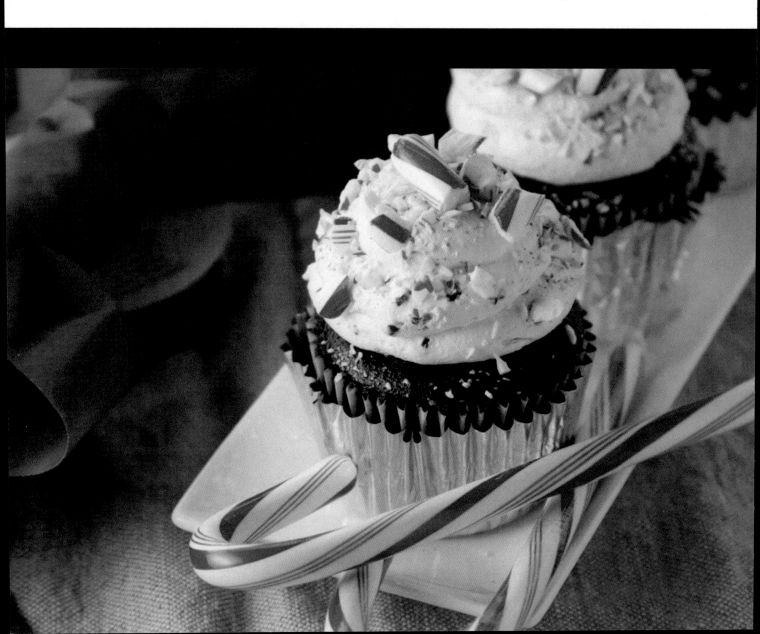

Directions

1. Preheat oven to 375°F. Prepare a muffin tin with 6 paper cups. Set aside.

2. In a medium bowl whisk the eggs with the coconut milk, xylitol, vanilla, peppermint extract and 3 tablespoons melted butter. Set aside.

3. In a small bowl whisk together the almond flour, SANE Cocoa Powder, baking powder and salt. Add to egg mixture whisking to incorporate all ingredients for about a minute. Pour into the 6 paper cups, place in the oven and bake until fully set in the center; about 15-18 minutes. When done, set on a wire rack to cool.

4. Make Frosting: In a small bowl, beat the coconut cream with an electric mixer until smooth. Add 1/4 cup softened butter and continue to beat another minute. Add the powdered erythritol; beat another minute then add peppermint extract and food coloring as desired (optional; red is pretty as pictured and green is festive with the red and white candies). Adjust for sweetness by adding a pinch of stevia if desired. Frost cupcakes using a piping bag or by hand. Sprinkle with crushed peppermint candies.

CHOCOLATE SWIRL ROLL

Total Time: 32 min
Prep: 20 min
Cook: 12 min

10 Servings
2 Whole-Food Fats Per Serving

Ingredients

- 1/3 second spray coconut oil
- 1 1/3 cups Xylitol
- 5 tbsps SANE Cocoa Powder
- 9 large Eggs (Whole)
- 2 tbsps Almond Flour
- 1/4 tsp Salt
- 1 1/3 cups Coconut Cream
- 2 ozs Unsweetened Baking Chocolate Squares
- 8 tbsps Unsalted Butter
- 1/4 tsp Vanilla Extract

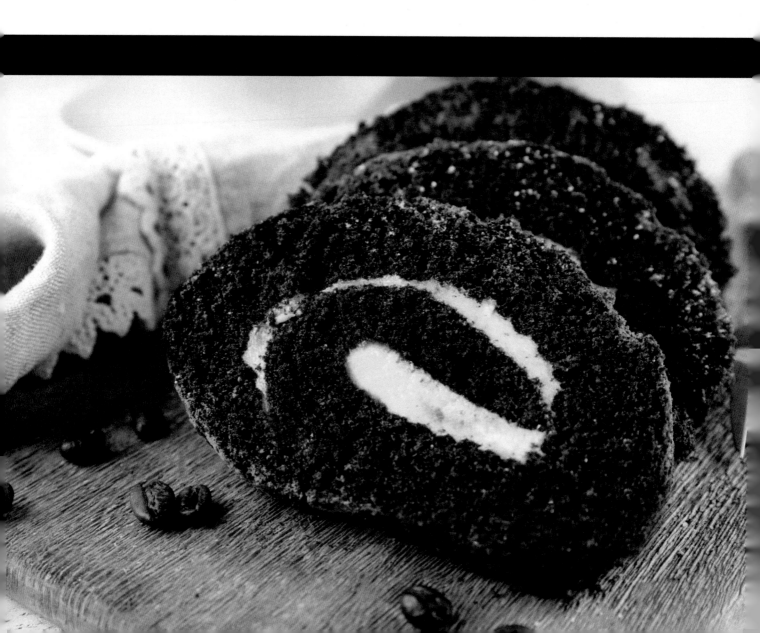

Directions

1. Preheat oven to 375°F. Spray a jellyroll pan with coconut oil spray; line with parchment, leaving a 2-inch border, spray again. Set aside. In a large bowl, whisk together 1 cup xylitol, 4 tbsps SANE Cocoa Powder and almond flour.

2. In another large bowl, beat egg yolks with an electric mixer on high speed until pale yellow and fluffy, about 3 minutes. Turn speed down to low and slowly mix in cocoa mixture until just combined. In another bowl, beat egg whites and salt with an electric mixer on high speed until stiff peaks form. Fold 1/3 of the whites into yolk mixture until just combined. Fold in remaining egg whites.

3. Spread batter evenly in prepared pan. Bake 15 minutes, until cake springs back when lightly touched and pulls away from sides of the pan. Cool cake in pan on wire rack for 30 minutes to 1 hour.

4. While cake is cooling, prepare filling and frosting. For the filling, whip 1 cup cream and 1 1/2 tablespoon xylitol in a medium bowl until stiff peaks form (do not overbeat). For the frosting, gradually combine 1/3 cup coconut cream and melted chocolate in a large bowl.

5. With an electric mixer on medium speed, beat in butter, 5 tablespoons xylitol, 1 tablespoon SANE Cocoa Powder and vanilla. Beat until smooth and fluffy, about 4 minutes. Chill in refrigerator until ready to use.

6. When cake is cool, slide cake from pan with parchment underneath. Place on counter top. Spread filling over cake, leaving a 1/2 inch border. Roll up cake from narrow end, using parchment to help.

7. Cut 1-inch diagonal pieces from each end. Transfer roll to a serving platter; place cut diagonal pieces on either side to form log stumps. Set aside.

8. To assemble: Use a generous dab of frosting to attach stumps to main log. Frost entire log, and run fork tines through frosting to create a bark-like texture.

Chocolate Walnut Cookies

Total Time: 26 min
Prep: 20 min
Cook: 6 min

32 Servings
1 Whole-Food Fat Per Serving

Ingredients

- 4 tbsps Almond Flour
- 1/8 tsp Baking Soda
- 3/4 cup Xylitol
- 1 1/2 ozs Unsweetened Baking Chocolate Squares

- 5 tbsps Coconut Cream
- 2 large Eggs (Whole)
- 2 tbsps Unsalted Butter
- 1 tsp Vanilla Extract
- 1/4 cup chopped English Walnuts

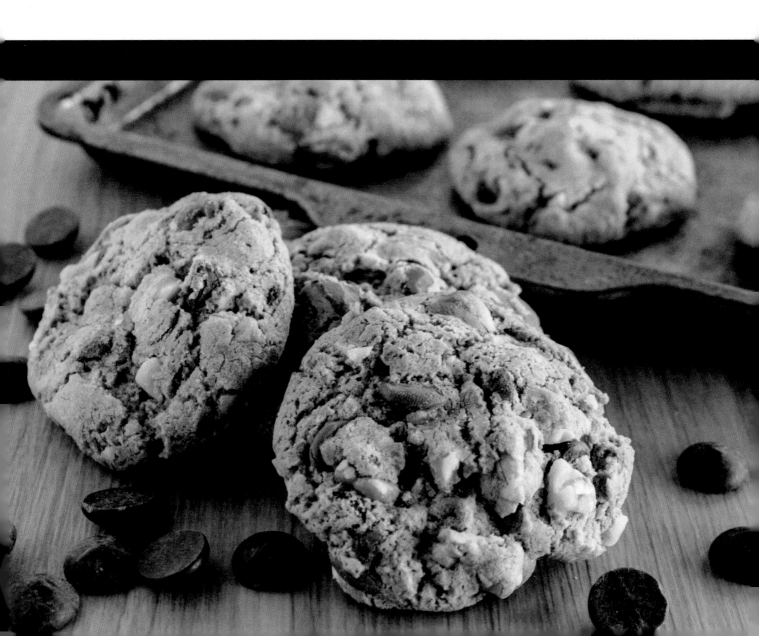

Directions

1. Preheat oven to 350°F. Lightly toast walnuts in an even layer on a cookie sheet for 6 to 8 minutes. Cool, coarsely chop the walnuts and set aside.

2. Put oven up to 375°F. Line two baking sheets with parchment paper or aluminum foil; set aside.

3. Whisk 4 tbsp almond flour and baking soda together in a bowl; set aside.

4. In the large bowl of an electric mixer, beat eggs and xylitol together on medium until light and slightly thickened. Place chocolate, coconut cream and butter in a microwavable bowl; microwave on medium until butter has melted and chocolate has softened (it need not be completely melted), 1 1/2 to 2 minutes. Let stand 5 minutes; stir until smooth.

5. Gradually beat the slightly warm chocolate mixture and vanilla extract into the egg mixture. Reduce speed to low, and beat in flour mixture, just until combined. Cover, and chill until thickened, 30 minutes.

6. Drop slightly rounded teaspoonfuls of dough, 1 inch apart, onto prepared sheet. Sprinkle tops of cookies with walnuts, lightly pressing into dough. Bake until cookies are just set but soft on top, 5 1/2 to 6 minutes. Cool cookies on baking sheet 1 minute before transferring to wire racks to cool completely. Store in an airtight container.

CHOCOLATE-COCONUT HAYSTACKS

Total Time: 27 min
Prep: 15 min
Cook: 12 min

6 Servings
1 Whole-Food Fat Per Serving

Ingredients

- 2 large Egg Whites
- 1 cup Xylitol
- 2 tbsps SANE Cocoa Powder
- 16 ozs Dried Coconut
- 2 tbsps Sugar Free Chocolate Syrup

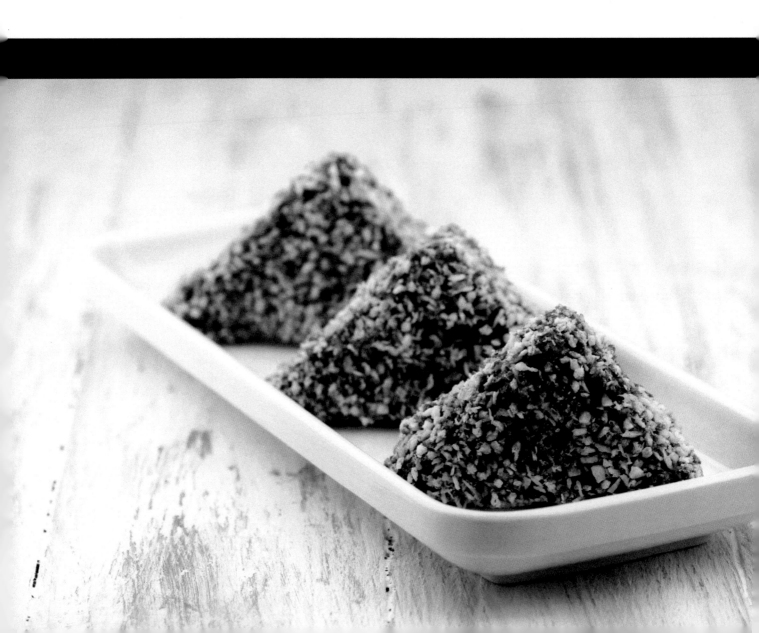

Directions

1. Heat oven to 325°F. Line baking sheets with aluminum foil.

2. Whip egg whites on low until medium peaks form; gradually beat in xylitol and SANE Cocoa Powder ; continue beating until stiff peaks form. Fold in coconut and syrup.

3. Drop mixture by rounded teaspoonfuls onto prepared baking sheets. Shape into little pyramids with wet fingertips. Bake 12 minutes. Cool on sheets 1 minute before transferring to wire racks to cool completely.

Note: Makes 32 Haystacks. 4 Haystacks = 1 serving

CHOCOLATE STRAWBERRIES

Total Time: 25 min
Prep: 25 min
Cook: 0 min

24 Servings
1 Whole-Food Fat Per Serving

Ingredients

- 8 ozs Sugar Free Chocolate Chips
- 24 large Strawberries

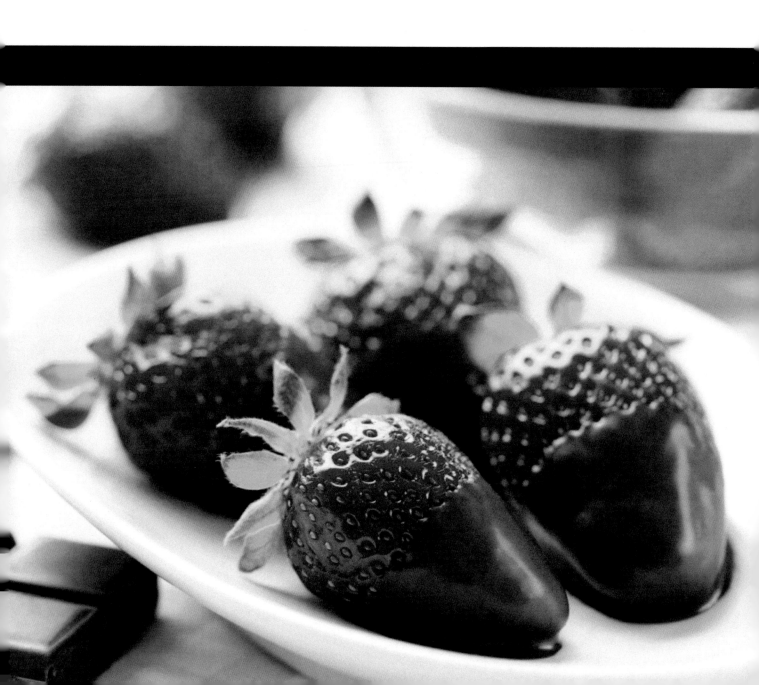

Directions

1. Line a baking sheet with aluminum foil or waxed paper. Break chocolate bars into pieces; place in the top part of a double boiler or a metal bowl set over (but not touching) a pot of simmering water. Stir one to two minutes, until chocolate is melted. Remove from heat.

2. Holding each strawberry by the stem, dip in chocolate, leaving a 1/4 inch border at the top. Gently shake off excess chocolate; place berry on foil. Repeat with remaining berries. Reheat chocolate if necessary.

3. Chill berries 40 minutes, until chocolate is set. May be prepared up to a day ahead.

Chocolate-Ginger Cake

Total Time: 1hr 5 min
Prep: 20 min
Cook: 45 min

16 Servings
1 Whole-Food Fat Per Serving

Ingredients

- 1/3 second Spray Coconut Oil
- 3/4 cup half Pecans
- 4 ozs Unsweetened Baking Chocolate Squares
- 1/3 cup Tap Water
- 1/3 cup Extra Virgin Coconut Oil
- 1/4 cup SANE Cocoa Powder
- 1/4 cup Almond Flour
- 2 1/4 cups Xylitol
- 12 large Eggs (Whole)
- 2 tsps Ginger (Ground)
- 1/4 tsp Coconut Cream

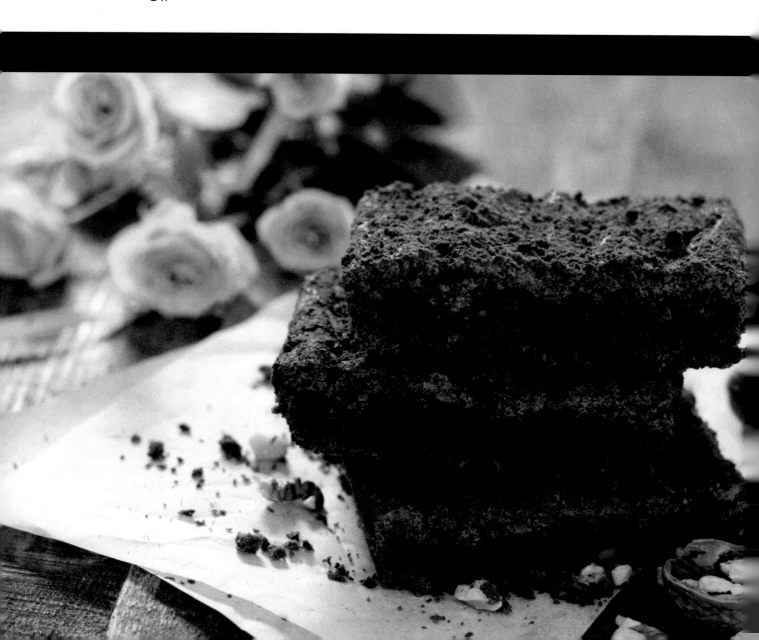

Directions

1. Preheat over to 350°F. Toast pecans in an even layer on a cookie sheet for 8 minutes. Cool, coarsely chop the pecans and set aside.

2. Lower oven to 325°F. Grease the bottom of a 10-inch tube pan, and line with parchment or waxed paper.

3. Place chocolate and the water in a microwavable bowl; microwave on high 1 to 2 minutes, until chocolate is melted, checking at 1-minute intervals. Stir until smooth, cool to lukewarm, then stir in oil; set aside.

4. In a food processor, pulse pecans, SANE Cocoa Powder and almond flour until pecans are finely ground. In a large bowl, beat egg yolks with cup xylitol on high speed with an electric mixer, until light and fluffy, about 5 minutes. Stir in melted chocolate, pecan mixture and ginger.

5. In another large bowl, beat egg whites and coconut cream on medium-high speed with an electric mixer, until frothy. Gradually add remaining xylitol, beating until stiff peaks form. With a rubber spatula, fold one-third of the meringue into the yolk mixture to lighten; fold in the remaining meringue until just combined.

6. Pour batter evenly in prepared pan and bake until a toothpick inserted in center of cake comes out clean, about 45 minutes. Allow cake to cool for 30 minutes before removing from pan.

7. To remove: Run a knife around the inner and outer rim of cake, place a wire rack or plate over pan, and invert. Remove pan, and peel off paper. Cool completely before cutting into 16 servings.

Chocolate-Mint Mousse Cake

Total Time: 3hr 25 min
Prep: 3hr
Cook: 25 min

8 Servings
4 Whole-Food Fats Per Serving

Ingredients

- 1/3 second Coconut Oil Cooking Spray
- 1 cup Coconut Cream
- 2 tsps Vanilla Extract
- 1/2 oz Coffee (Instant Powder)
- 1 1/4 cup Almond Flour
- 1/2 cup SANE Cocoa Powder

- 1/2 cup half Pecans
- 1/2 tsp Baking Powder
- 1/2 tsp Salt
- 1 cup Unsalted Butter
- 1 cup Xylitol
- 8 servings SANE Chocolate Mint Mousse
- 4 large Eggs (Whole)

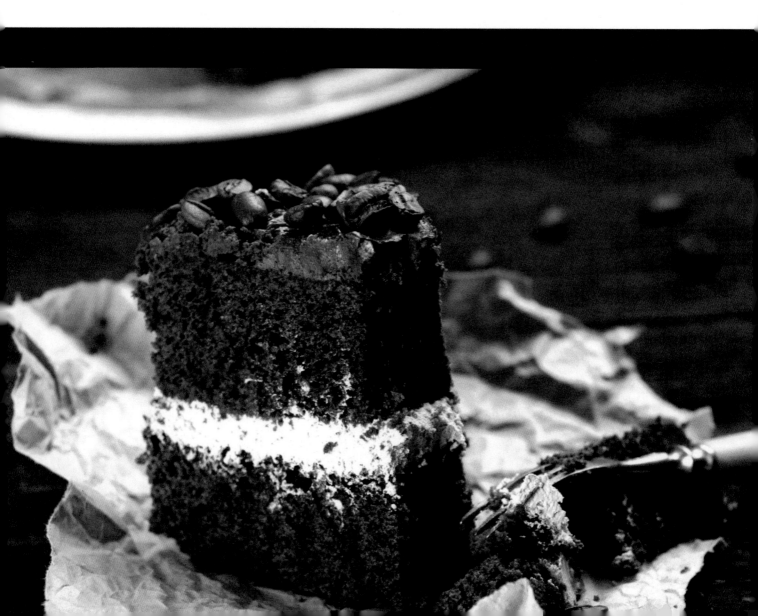

Directions

1. Use the SANE Chocolate-Mint Mousse.

2. Preheat oven to 325°F. Grease two 8 round cake pans with coconut oil spray.

3. In a small bowl, mix coconut cream, vanilla and coffee. Set aside. In a medium bowl, whisk together almond flour, SANE cocoa powder, pecans, baking powder and salt. Set aside. In a large bowl, with an electric mixer on medium speed, beat butter with half of the xylitol until light and fluffy, about 5 minutes. Separate the eggs into yolks and whites. Add egg yolks, one at a time, beating well and scraping down the sides of the bowl after each addition. Add heavy cream mixture and beat until well-blended. Turn mixer speed down to low, and slowly add dry ingredients, one third at a time, beating until just-combined. Set aside.

4. In another large bowl, beat egg whites until soft peaks form, about 3 minutes. Add remaining xylitol and beat until stiff peaks, about 1 more minute. Using a rubber spatula, fold whites into chocolate batter in three parts, combining thoroughly after each addition.

5. Divide batter in prepared pans; smooth tops. Bake 20 minutes, or until cake springs back when touched in the middle. Cool in pans on racks 5 minutes; invert onto racks to cool completely, about 2 hours.

6. To assemble cake: Cut off rounded tops of each cake. Place one cake layer on a serving plate, cut side down. Spread top with half of mousse filling, leaving a 1/2 border. Place cut side of the other cake layer down on top of the mousse, pressing gently, being careful not to let mousse squirt out. Top this with remaining mousse and swirl decoratively. Garnish with raspberries and mint leaves. Makes 8 servings.

CINNAMON CUSTARD

Total Time: 50 min
Prep: 20 min
Cook: 30 min

6 Servings
3 Whole-Food Fats Per Serving

Ingredients

- 2 cups Coconut Cream
- 1/2 tsp Cinnamon
- 2 large Eggs (Whole)
- 1/2 cup Xylitol

- 1/8 tsp Salt
- 1/2 tsp Vanilla Extract
- 6 tbsps Caramel Sugar Free Syrup
- 2 large Egg Yolks

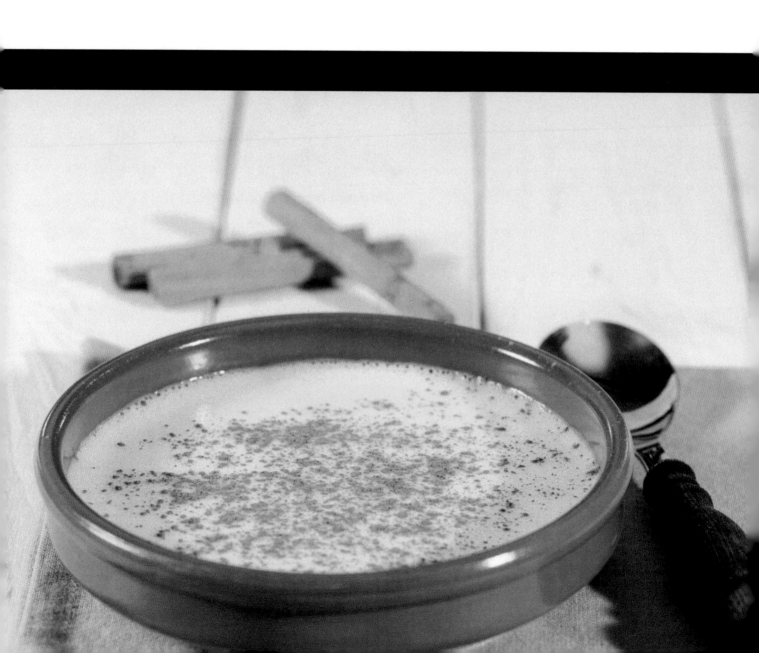

Directions

1. In a medium-size heavy saucepan, combine cream and cinnamon. Heat over medium heat, whisking constantly to thoroughly blend cinnamon into coconut cream, just until cream begins to steam. Do not boil. Remove from heat.

2. Heat oven to 300°F.

3. In a medium bowl, whisk eggs, egg yolks, xylitol and salt together until pale yellow and slightly thickened.

4. Using a soup ladle and whisking constantly, very gradually pour in the hot cream. When all the cream has been added, whisk in the vanilla extract.

5. Pour about 1/2 cup of the cream mixture into each of six 4-ounce custard cups (or pour entire mixture into a 2-quart round baking dish).

6. Place the cups or baking dish in a roasting pan. Carefully pour enough boiling water (about 4 cups) in the roasting pan to come halfway up the sides of the cups or baking dish.

7. Bake until custard is still slightly loose in center, about 30 minutes. (Bake the baking dish about 5 minutes more).

8. Using an oven mitt, carefully remove cups from water bath.

9. Serve warm, at room temperature or cold, toping each serving with 1 tablespoon of a caramel sugar free syrup.

Cinnamon-Almond Meringues

Total Time: 3hr 30 min   8 Servings
Prep: 2hr   1 Whole-Food Fat Per Serving
Cook: 1hr 30 min

Ingredients

- 1/2 cup whole Almonds
- 4 TBSP Xylitol
- 3 large Egg Whites

- 1/2 tsp Pure Almond Extract
- 1/2 tsp Cinnamon
- 1/8 tsp Coconut Cream

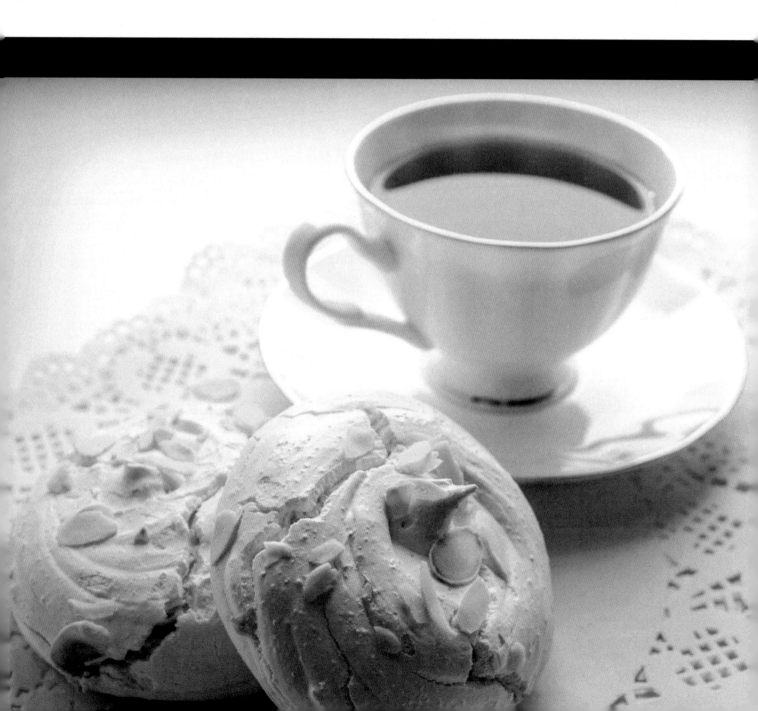

Directions

1. Heat oven to 200°F. Line a baking sheet with aluminum foil.

2. In a food processor, chop nuts with xylitol until nuts are finely ground.

3. In a large bowl, with electric mixer at high speed, beat egg whites until soft peaks form. Add the coconut cream, almond extract and cinnamon beating until stiff peaks form. Gently fold in nut mixture.

4. With a spoon, drop 8 evenly spaced mounds onto prepared baking sheet. Make a depression in center of each with the back of the spoon. Bake meringues on center oven rack 1 1/2 hours, until golden and very dry. Turn off oven and let meringues dry in oven until cool. Carefully peel meringues off foil.

Classic Apple Tart

Total Time: 1hr 15 min   8 Servings
Prep: 30 min   1 Whole-Food Fat Per Serving
Cook: 45 min

Ingredients

- 5 medium (2-3/4″ diameter) (~3 per lb) Apples
- 1/4 cup Xylitol
- 3/4 tsp Cinnamon
- 1/8 tsp Nutmeg (Ground)
- 1 serving SANE Pie Crust
- 1 tbsp Unsalted Butter

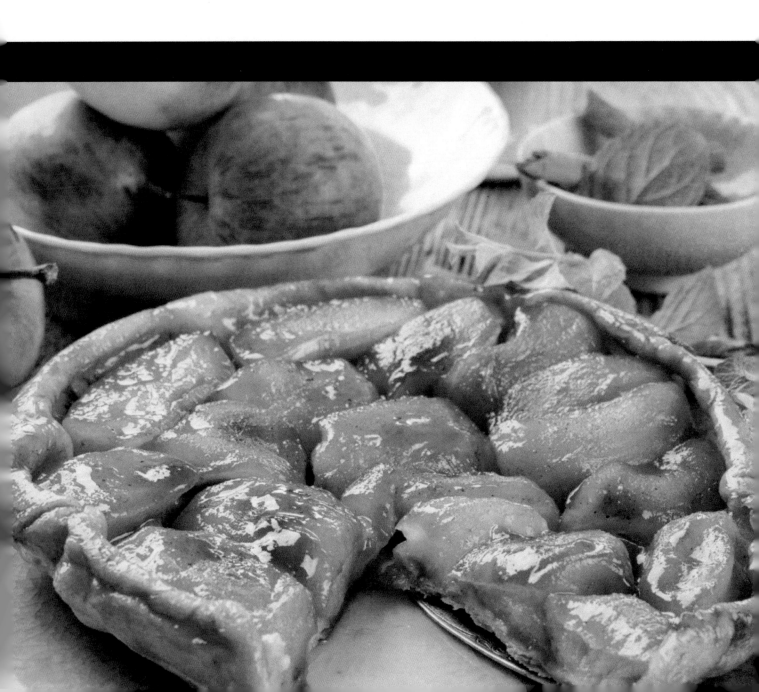

Directions

1. Prepare SANE Pie Crust and press evenly into a 10-inch tart pan with removable bottom. Freeze 15 minutes.

2. Heat oven to 350°F. In a large bowl, combine apples, xylitol cinnamon and nutmeg. Toss until apples are evenly coated. Spoon into crust; dot top with butter.

3. Bake tart 30 minutes. Cover loosely with foil and bake 10 to 20 minutes more, until apples are tender when pierced with the tip of a knife. Cool tart on wire rack.

4. Serve warm or at room temperature, with ice cream and praline sauce, if desired.

Coconut Cookies

Total Time: 33 min
Prep: 8 min
Cook: 27 min

12 Servings
1 Whole-Food Fat Per Serving

Ingredients

- 1/3 second Spray Coconut Oil
- 1/2 cup Almond flour
- 1/3 cup Dried Coconut
- 1/4 cup whole Hazelnuts or Filberts
- 2 large Egg Whites
- 1/8 can Seltzer Water

- 1 1/2 tsps Coconut Extract
- 1/2 tsp Vanilla Extract
- 1/2 tsp Salt
- 8 tbsps Unsalted Butter
- 7 tbsps Xylitol

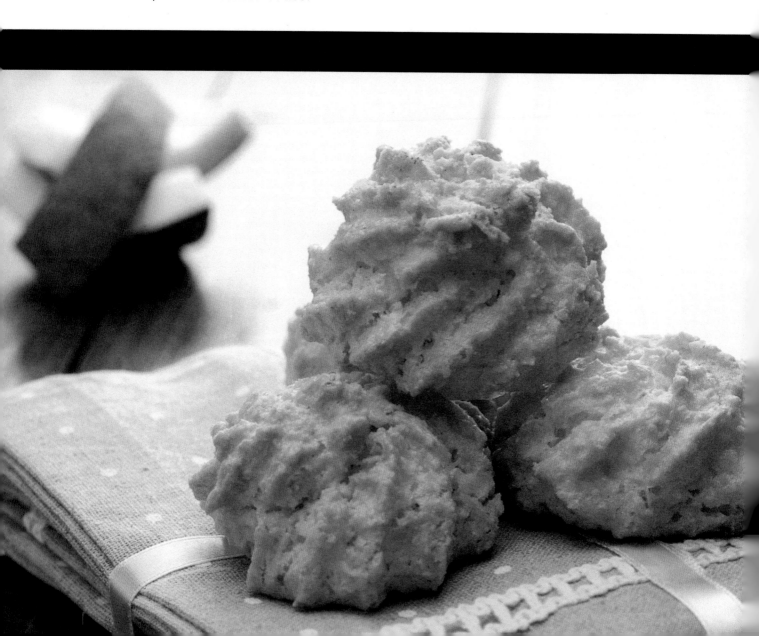

Directions

1. Preheat oven to 350°F. Toast hazelnuts in an even layer on a cookie sheet for 8 minutes. Cool, coarsely chop and set aside.

2. Increase oven temperature to 375°F. Grease baking sheet with spray coconut oil.

3. In large bowl, combine almond flour, unsweetened coconut, hazelnuts, egg whites, 2 Tbsp seltzer, 1 1/2 tsp coconut and 1/2 tsp vanilla extract., salt, butter and xylitol. Mix well.

4. Drop by rounded 1 tablespoonful (12 cookies) onto prepared baking sheet. Bake 20 minutes, or until light golden brown. Cool cookies on baking sheet 1 minute before transferring to wire racks to cool completely.

Coconut Doughnuts

Total Time: 30 min
Prep: 5 min
Cook: 25 min

6 Servings
1 Whole-Food Fat Per Serving

Ingredients

- 1/2 cup of Coconut Flour
- 1/4 teaspoon of sea salt
- 1/4 teaspoon of baking soda

- 6 eggs
- 1/2 cup SANE honey
- 1 tablespoon of Vanilla
- 1/2 cup of Extra Virgin Coconut Oil

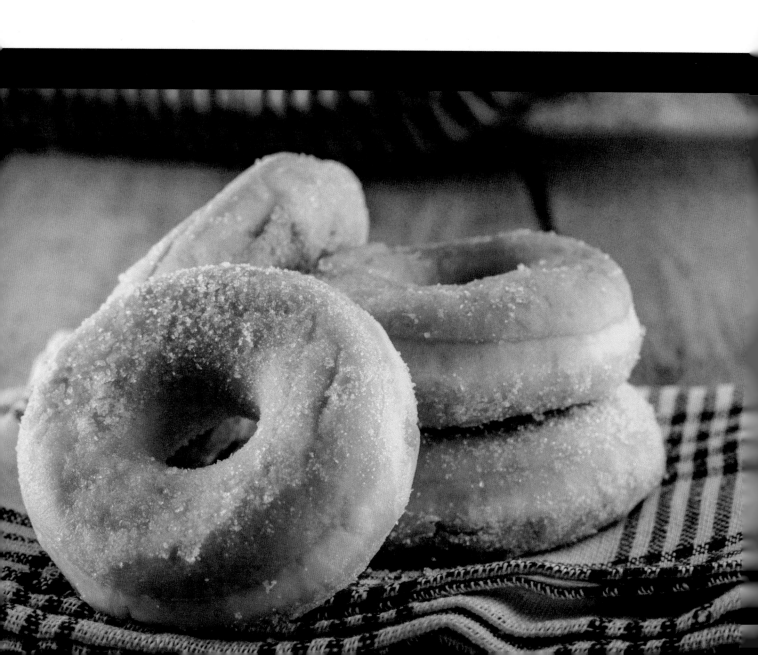

Directions

1. Preheat oven to 350 degrees F.

2. Blend all the dry ingredients together in a bowl.

3. Using a whisk, or mixer on a low setting, blend in all the wet ingredients into the dry ingredients.

4. Mix until well-blended.

5. Fill donut pan circles about 2/3 of the way full with batter.

6. Bake for about 20 minutes, or until a toothpick comes out clean.

Honey-dipped, toasted coconut topping

1. Warm a few tablespoons of SANE honey in a saucer (You can put it in the microwave for about 10 seconds).

2. Toast some coconut flakes for about 5 minutes at 300 degrees F.

3. Dip each donut in the honey and then in the toasted coconut.

Coconut Layer Cake

Total Time: 52 min
Prep: 30 min
Cook: 22 min

12 Servings
3 Whole-Food Fats Per Serving

Ingredients

- 8 large Eggs (Whole)
- 1 1/2 cups Xylitol
- 3 tsps Coconut Extract
- 2/3 cup Almond Flour

- 1 tsp Baking Powder
- 6 large Egg Whites
- 2 cups Unsalted Butter
- 1/4 tsp Salt
- 2/3 cup Dried Coconut

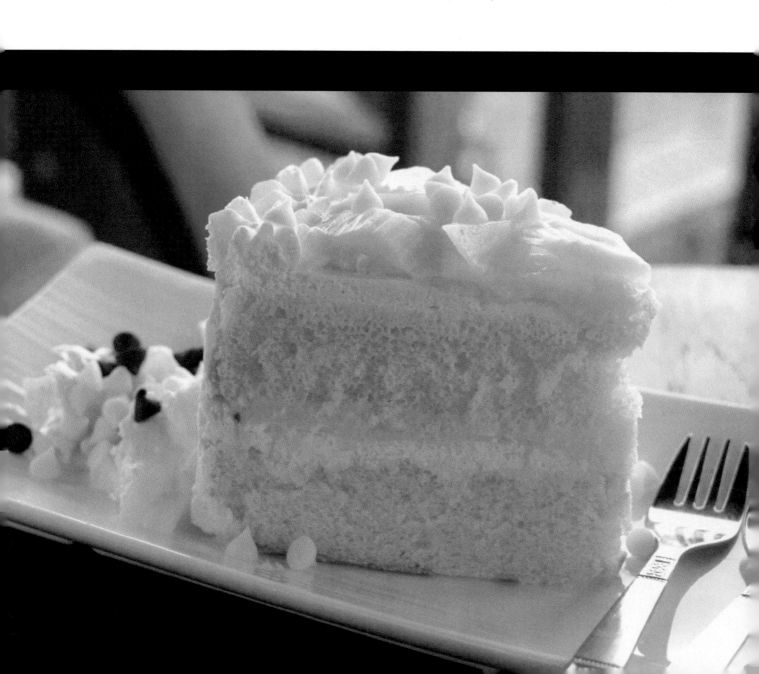

Directions

1. Heat oven to 350°F. Grease two 8-inch cake pans; line bottoms with parchment paper; then grease the paper.

2. With an electric mixer on high, beat whole eggs, 3/4 cup xylitol and 1 tbsp coconut extract until ribbons form, about 5 minutes.

3. In three additions cup sift almond flour, baking powder and salt over egg mixture; fold in with a rubber spatula to combine.

4. Fold in 1/2 cup melted butter. Then pour batter into prepared pans.

5. Bake for 22 minutes until cake springs back in middle when lightly touched. Cool in pans on wire racks 5 minutes. Line racks with paper towels and invert cake layers. Gently peel off parchment and cool completely.

6. For frosting: in a double boiler or a bowl placed over simmering water, whisk egg whites, 3/4 cup xylitol and salt until temperature reaches 130°F. Transfer whites to mixing bowl and beat on high speed until cool and fully whipped. Reduce speed to medium and beat in 1 1/2 cups room temperature butter 1 tablespoon at a time until well combined, thick and creamy, about 10 minutes – do not rush the process.

7. Place one cake layer on serving plate. Mix 1 cup frosting with half the coconut (1/3 cup); frost bottom layer. Place top cake layer over bottom layer. Cover top and sides with remaining frosting and pat remaining 1/3 cup coconut over frosting. Optional: toast coconut (3-5 minutes at 350°F). Makes 12 servings.

Coconut Macaroons

Total Time: 32 min   30 Servings
Prep: 20 min   1 Whole-Food Fat Per Serving
Cook: 12 min

Ingredients

- 1/3 second Spray Coconut Oil
- 4 large Egg Whites
- 2/3 cup Xylitol
- 1/2 tsp Vanilla Extract
- 1/4 tsp Salt
- 2 cups Dried Coconut

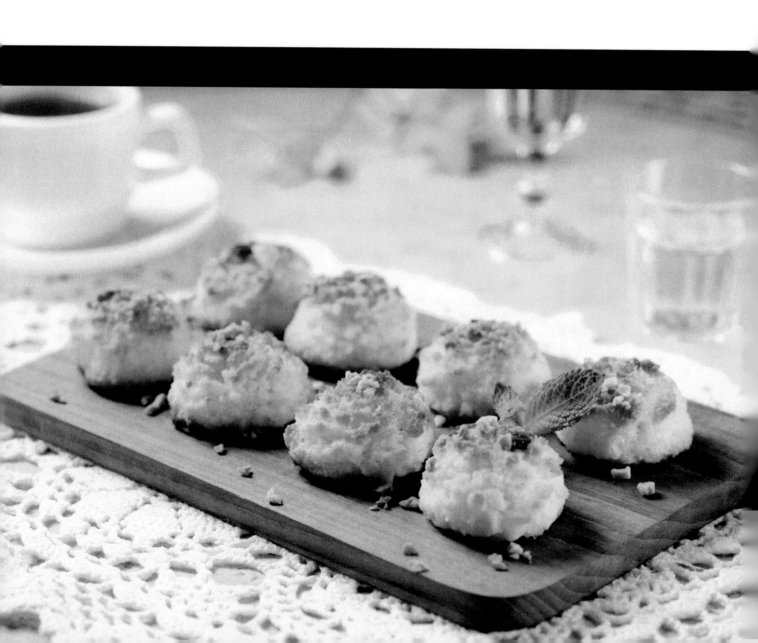

Directions

1. Heat oven to 325°F. Spray two baking sheets with spray coconut oil.

2. With an electric mixer on medium speed, beat egg whites until medium peaks form. Gradually beat in xylitol, vanilla extract and salt. Turn speed up to high and continue beating until stiff (but not dry) peaks form.

3. Using a rubber spatula, fold in coconut.

4. Drop tablespoon-sized mounds of mixture onto prepared baking sheets. Bake 15 minutes. Cool on sheets 1 minute before carefully transferring to wire racks to cool completely.

Coco-Coconut Cashew Truffles

Total Time: 3hr
Prep: 3hr
Cook: 0 min

32 Servings
1 Whole-Food Fat Per Serving

Ingredients

- 3/4 cup Coconut Cream
- 2 tbsps Xylitol
- 2 tbsps Unsalted Butter Stick

- 17 ozs Unsweetened Baking Chocolate Squares
- 3/4 tsp Vanilla Extract
- 8 ozs Dried Coconut
- 1/2 cup Organic Raw Cashews

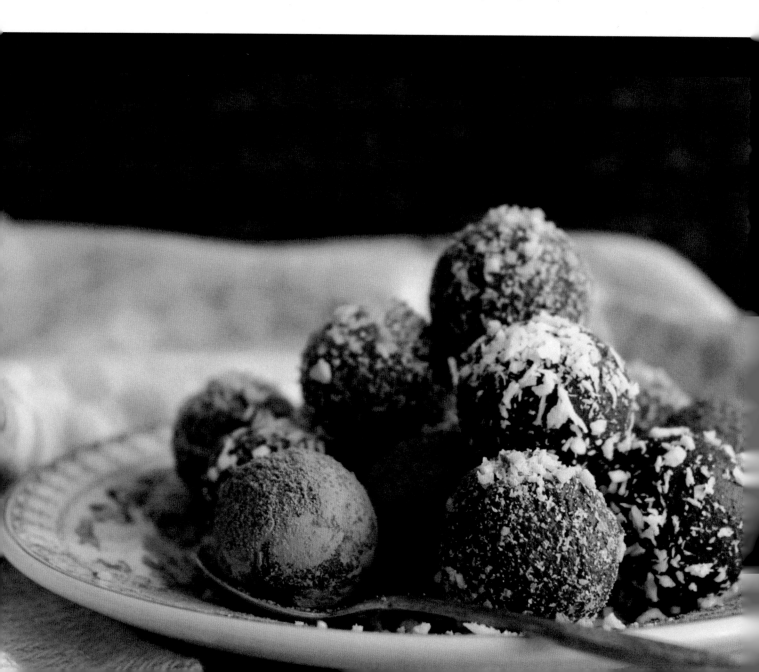

Directions

1. Combine coconut cream, xylitol and butter in a small saucepan. Bring to a simmer. Place chopped chocolate in a medium bowl; pour hot cream mixture over chocolate. Let stand 5 minutes.

2. Stir chocolate mixture gently until chocolate is completely melted. Stir in extract and 1/2 cup of the coconut. Refrigerate until firm, about 1 hour 45 minutes, stirring occasionally (Truffles will be easier to form if the mixture is not too stiff).

3. Toast the remaining 1/2 cup coconut in a dry skillet over medium heat, shaking often, until lightly browned; transfer to a bowl and cool.

4. Roll the chocolate mixture into 32 balls about the size of large marbles. Roll half of the balls in cashews and half in toasted coconut. Place in an airtight container between layers of wax paper. Can refrigerate up to one week.

Coconut-Lime Mousse

Total Time: 10 min
Prep: 10 min
Cook: 0 min

4 Servings
2 Whole-Food Fats Per Serving

Ingredients

- 1 1/4 cup Coconut Cream
- 8 tsps Xylitol
- 1/4 cup Fresh Lime Juice
- 1 tsp Vanilla Extract

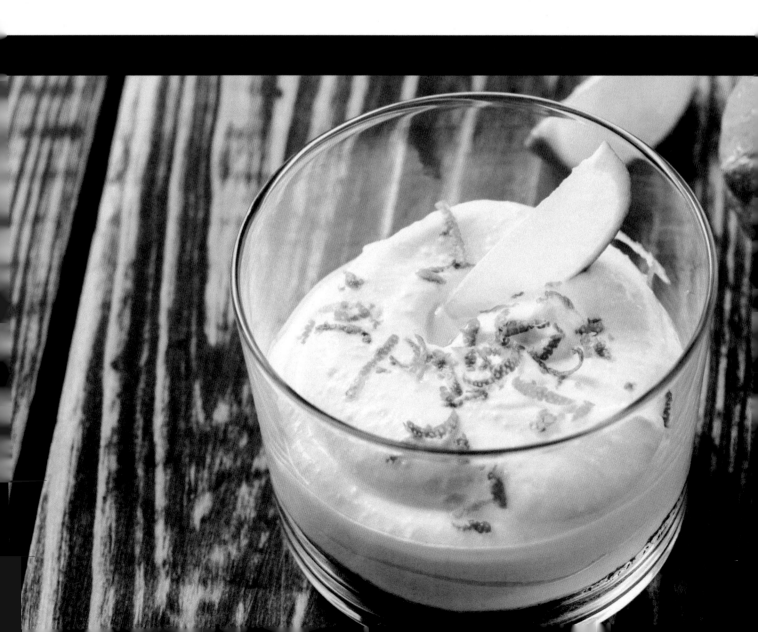

Directions

1. Using an electric mixer, beat together 2 oz coconut cream and xylitol until smooth.

2. Slowly add 1/4 cup lime juice, beating until creamy.

3. Beat in 1 teaspoon coconut extract (vanilla may be used if coconut is unavailable) and 1 cup coconut cream until fluffy.

4. Place in four bowls, sprinkle with 1 Tbsp unsweetened coconut flakes each and refrigerate until serving.

DARK MOCHA PUDDING

Total Time: 20 min
Prep: 10 min
Cook: 10 min

8 Servings
1 Whole-Food Fat Per Serving

Ingredients

- 2 cups Organic Coconut Milk
- 1/2 cup Coconut Cream
- 1/8 tsp Salt
- 1/3 rounded cup Erythritol
- 2 large Egg Yolks

- 1 tsp dry Coffee (Instant Powder)
- 1/2 tsp Thick-It-Up
- 1 tsp Vanilla Extract
- 1 tbsp Unsalted Butter
- 1 tbsp SANE Cocoa Powder
- 2 ozs Sugar Free Chocolate Chips

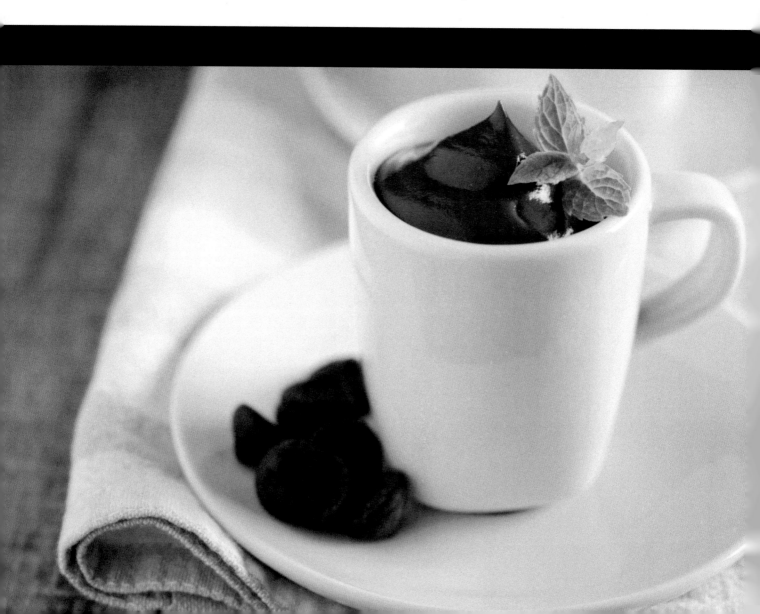

Directions

1. Place 1 3/4 cups of the coconut milk in a sauce pan with the coconut cream, salt and erythritol. Bring to a simmer over medium heat.

2. While the milk is heating, whisk the egg yolks with the remaining 1/4 cup coconut milk and instant coffee. Once the milk mixture is hot pour a steady stream in the egg yolks while whisking to temper them. Once all the milk has been incorporated pour the mixture back into the sauce pan over medium heat.

3. While it is heating back up, quickly whisk together the SANE cocoa powder and Thick-It-Up in a small bowl then whisk it into the milk and egg mixture. Cook and stir pudding continuously to be sure the egg does not curdle.

4. Cook until it begins to thicken (mixture will still be slightly runny); about 2-3 minutes. Do not allow pudding to boil. Take off the heat once thickened; about 3-5 minutes.

5. Melt the chocolate with the butter in small bowl in a microwave at 30 second intervals. Do not overheat. Stir to blend and then scrape into the hot pudding stirring to blend completely. Remove from heat.

6. Cool quickly over an ice water bath; place plastic wrap on the surface to prevent a skin from forming. Once cooled place in the refrigerator to continue cooling or immediately dish into serving bowls, top with coconut cream if desired and serve.

7. Makes 2 2/3 cups. Each serving is 1/3 cup. This pudding is very rich, consider serving it in a small glass dish layered with coconut cream.

DECADENT BROWNIES

Total Time: 1hr 10 min
Prep: 10 min
Cook: 1hr

16 brownies
1 Whole-Food Fat Per Serving

Ingredients

- 1/2 cup Coconut flour
- 1/2 cup SANE Cocoa Powder
- 1/2 cup butter, melted

- 3 eggs
- 1/2 cup SANE honey
- 1 tsp. vanilla extract

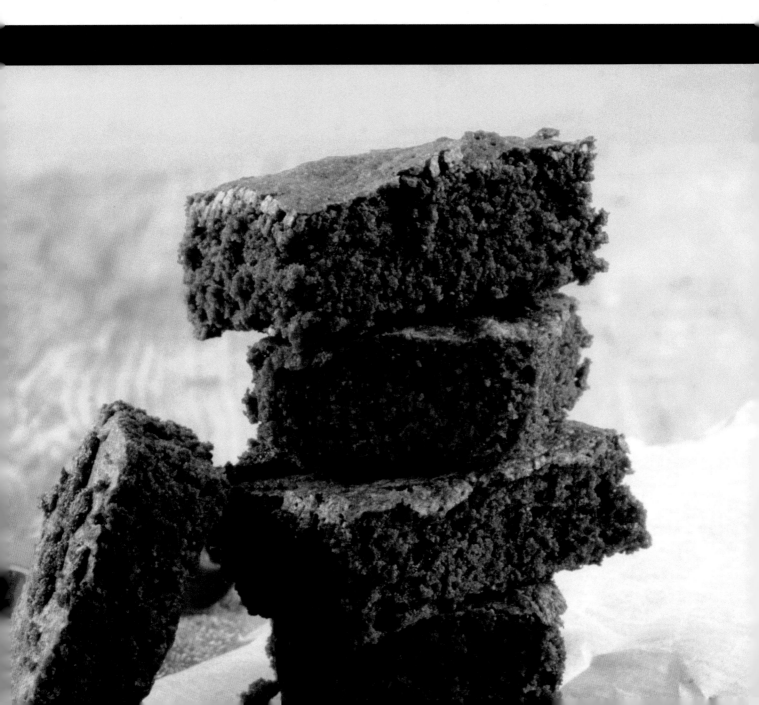

Directions

1. Preheat the oven to 300 and grease a glass baking dish (8×8 or 9×9).

2. Mix together all ingredients.

3. Pour into the baking dish and bake for 30-35 minutes, until a toothpick inserted into the center comes out clean. Cool for 30 minutes before cutting or removing from the pan.

4. These store well at room temperature or in the fridge for a few days. Make sure you keep them in an airtight container.

DECADENT CHOCOLATE CAKE

Total Time: 1hr
Prep: 15 min
Cook: 45 min

12 Servings
1 Whole-Food Fat Per Serving

Ingredients

- 4 ozs Unsweetened Baking Chocolate Squares
- 1/2 cup Unsalted Butter
- 1 tbsp Tap Water

- 3/4 cup Xylitol
- 2 tbsps SANE Cocoa Powder
- 1 tsp Vanilla Extract
- 6 large Eggs (Whole)

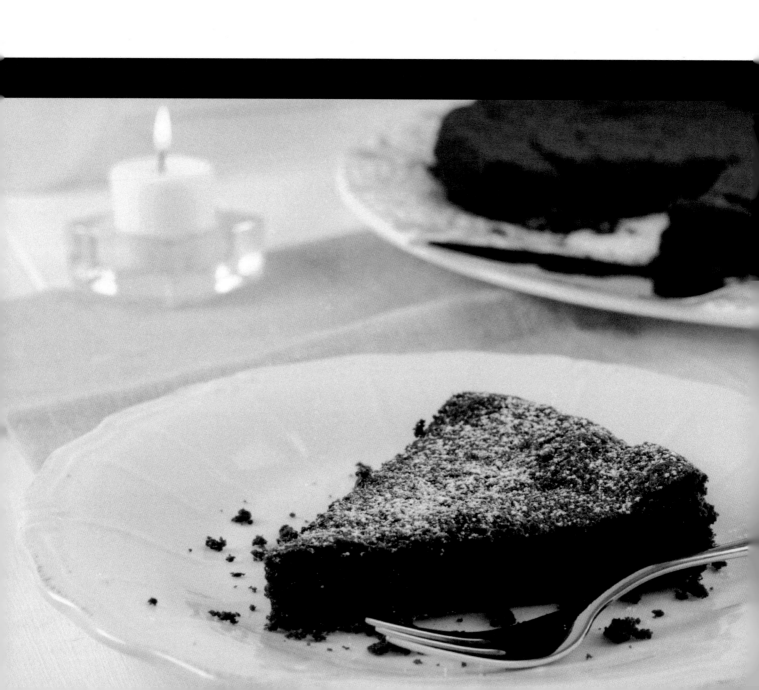

Directions

1. Heat oven to 325°F. Grease an 8-inch spring form pan and line the bottom with parchment paper; grease paper and set aside.

2. Melt chocolate, butter and water in the top of a double boiler set over simmering water, stirring to combine. Remove from heat and transfer to a large bowl; cool to room temperature. Add ¼ cup of the xylitol, SANE cocoa powder and vanilla extract to chocolate mixture, stirring until combined.

3. In a medium bowl, with an electric mixer on medium-high, beat eggs until mixture forms thick ribbons when beater is lifted, about 6 minutes. Reduce speed to medium; gradually add remaining ½ cup xylitol and beat until combined, 1 minute. Stir one-third of the egg mixture into the chocolate mixture to lighten. In two additions, fold in remaining egg mixture until well combined.

4. Pour batter into prepared pan, smoothing top. Bake until evenly risen and almost set, 40-45 minutes (it will look like a brownie). Cool completely on a wire rack. To serve, run a knife around edge of pan and remove rim. Cut into 12 pieces and serve with coconut cream (optional).

Espresso Chocolate Cake

Total Time: 1hr
Prep: 25 min
Cook: 35 min

8 Servings
2 Whole-Food Fats Per Serving

Ingredients

- 10 ozs Sugar Free Chocolate Chips
- 10 tbsps Unsalted Butter
- 1 tsp rounded Coffee (Instant Powder, Decaffeinated)
- 1 tbsp Tap Water
- 1 tsp Vanilla Extract
- 1/4 tsp Salt
- 24 tsps Erythritol
- 1 pinch Stevia
- 4 large Eggs (Whole)
- 1/3 cup SANE Cocoa Powder

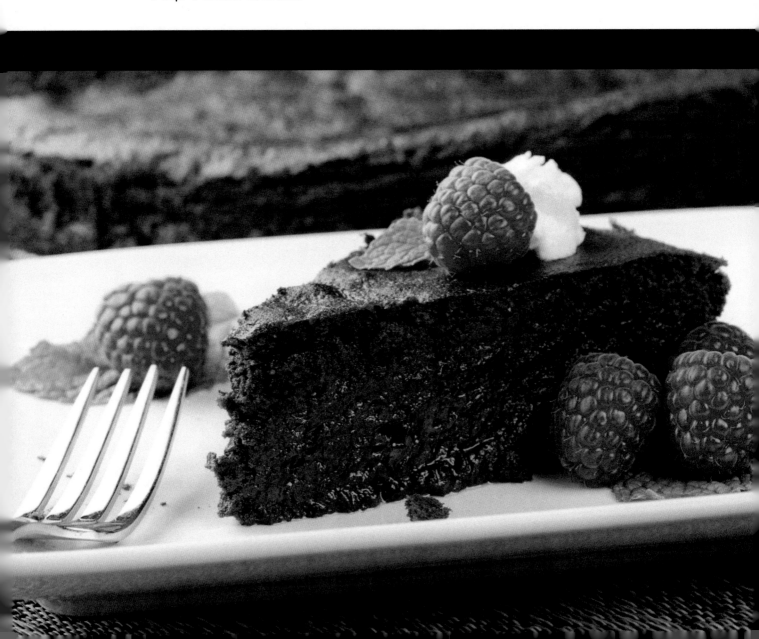

Directions

1. Preheat oven to 325°F. Grease an 8-inch round baking pan and line with parchment paper (a spring form pan works best). Set aside.

2. Melt chocolate and butter in a double boiler. Remove from heat and transfer to a large bowl. Alternatively melt chocolate with butter in a small bowl in the microwave at 30 second intervals; stirring in between. In a small cup, mix espresso powder, water, vanilla and salt; stir into chocolate. Set mixture aside to cool.

3. With an electric mixer on medium-high speed, beat eggs, 1/2 cup (24 tsp) erythritol, stevia and SANE Cocoa Powder until it falls in thick ribbons when the beater is lifted, about 6 minutes. In three additions, fold eggs into the chocolate mixture.

4. Pour batter into prepared pan and smooth top. Bake 30-35 minutes, or until a toothpick inserted near middle of cake comes out with a few moist crumbs and cake is evenly raised. Cool completely on a wire rack. To remove cake, run a knife around edge of pan. Dip bottom of pan into hot water for 1 minute, then turn cake out onto cutting board. (if using a spring form pan, carefully remove sides and serve on the platter.) Turn right side up onto a serving platter. Serve with coconut cream and raspberries, if desired.

FROZEN CHOCOLATE FUDGE TART

Total Time: 3hr 50 min   12 Servings
Prep: 3hr 30 min   2 Whole-Food Fats Per Serving
Cook: 20 min

Ingredients

- 5 tbsps SANE Cocoa Powder
- 1/2 tsp Cinnamon
- 7 tbsps Xylitol
- 4 tbsps Unsalted Butter
- 3 cups Coconut Cream

- 4 ozs Sugar Free Chocolate Chips
- 2 tsps Vanilla Extract
- 1 2/3 servings All Purpose SANE Baking Mix
- 1 tsp dry Coffee (Instant Powder)

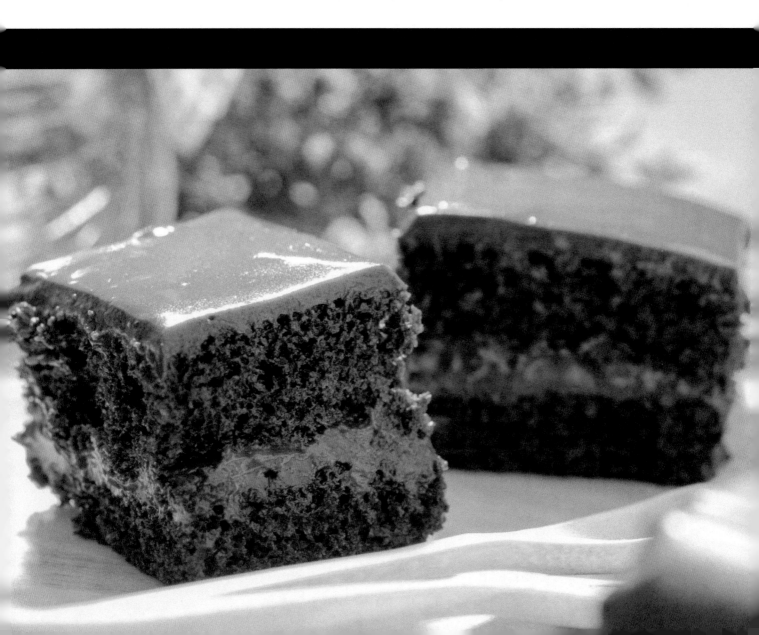

Directions

1. Preheat oven to 425°F.

2. For the crust: In a food processor, pulse the 1/2 cup All Purpose SANE Baking Mix, 4 tablespoons SANE Cocoa Powder, cinnamon and 3 tablespoons xylitol to combine, about 10 seconds. Add cold chopped butter and pulse until mixture resembles a coarse meal, about 30 seconds. Add 1/2 cup coconut cream and pulse until mixture begins to come together, about 30 more seconds.

3. Transfer dough to a 9-inch pie plate and pat into an even layer on bottom and sides. Prick the dough about 15 times with a fork and crimp edges decoratively. Cover lightly with aluminum foil and bake 10 minutes, until set. Uncover and bake 10 more minutes until light golden brown. Cool crust before filling.

4. For the filling: Place chocolate and 1 teaspoon vanilla extract in a medium bowl. Heat one cup coconut cream and instant coffee over medium-high heat until just about to boil, about 4 minutes. Pour over chocolate, let stand 3 minutes, then stir until chocolate is melted. Pour into pie shell, smooth top and chill 30 minutes.

5. In a medium bowl with an electric mixer on high speed, beat remaining coconut cream, 4 tablespoons xylitol, 1 teaspoon vanilla extract and 1 tablespoon SANE Cocoa Powder until medium peaks form, about 4 minutes. Spread over chocolate layer and freeze at least 2.5 hours or until firm. Remove from freezer 10 minutes before serving.

MEXICAN HOT CHOCOLATE SOUFFLÉ

Total Time: 32 min   2 Servings
Prep: 15 min   1 Whole-Food Fat Per Serving
Cook: 17 min

Ingredients

- 1 tsp Unsalted Butter
- 9 tsps Erythritol
- 4 tbsps Sugar Free Chocolate Chips
- 2 large Egg Yolks
- 1/2 fl oz Tap Water
- 1 tsp Vanilla Extract
- 3/4 tsp Cinnamon
- 1/8 tbsp Red or Cayenne Pepper
- 3 large Egg Whites
- 1 pinch Stevia

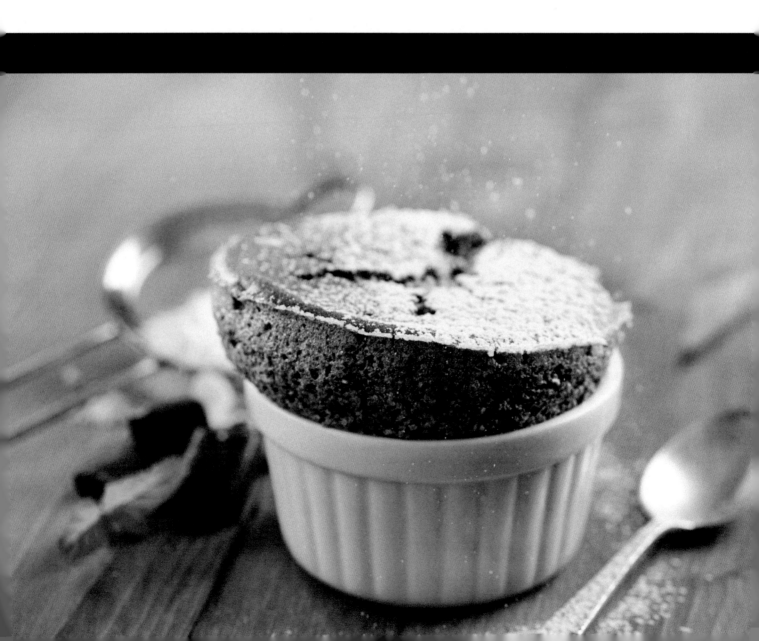

Directions

1. Preheat oven to 400°F. Grease the bottom and up the sides of a 2-cup deep soufflé dish with butter and sprinkle 1 ½ teaspoons erythritol to coat all buttered areas. Set aside.

2. Melt the chocolate in a small bowl in a microwave at 30 second intervals until melted through. Do not overheat and stir between intervals.

3. In a medium bowl whisk 2 egg yolks with 1 tablespoon warm water, 1 teaspoon vanilla, 3/4 teaspoon ground cinnamon and 1/8 teaspoon cayenne pepper (add more if more spice is desired). Add the melted chocolate and whisk until incorporated and smooth. Set aside.

4. In a medium bowl whip the egg whites with 2 ½ tablespoons erythritol and a large pinch of stevia to stiff peaks. Whisk a few tablespoons of the egg whites into the chocolate mixture, then quickly but gently fold in the remaining egg whites until a lighter airy mixture results and all ingredients are blended (do not over blend or you will deflate the egg whites).

5. Pour into the souffle dish and bake on a sheet pan for 15-18 minutes. The souffle will rise over the top of the dish and it should appear slightly jiggly but not wet in the center when shaken. Serve immediately.

MINI CHOCOLATE CHIP MUFFINS

Total Time: 25 min
Prep: 10 min
Cook: 15 min

24 Servings
1 Whole-Food Fat Per Serving

Ingredients

- 1 cup Almond Flour
- 1 tsp Baking Powder
- 1/2 cup Xylitol
- 1/4 tsp Salt

- 10 tbsps Coconut Cream
- 2 tbsps Unsalted Butter
- 1 fl oz Tap Water
- 2 tsps Vanilla Extract
- 4 ozs SANE Chocolate Chips

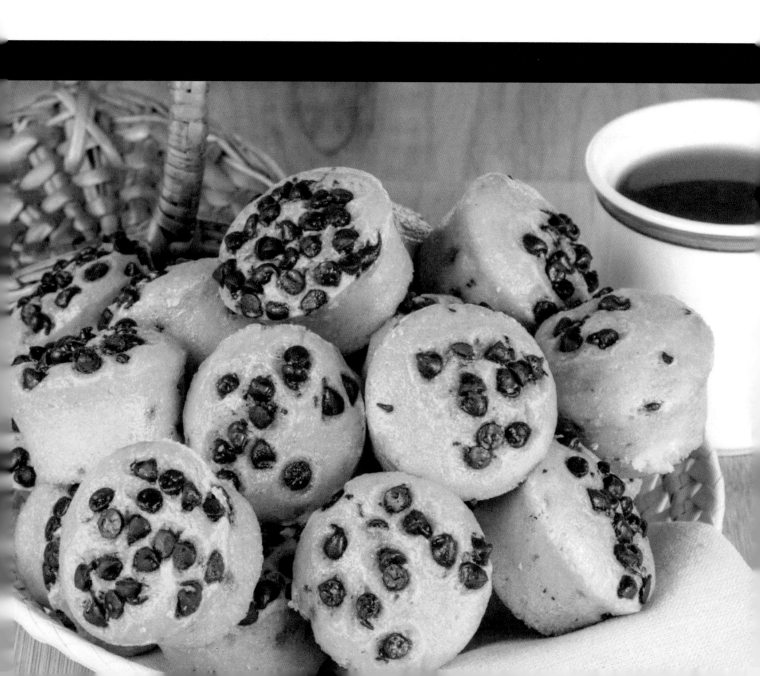

Directions

1. Heat oven to 350°F. Grease two 12-compartment mini muffin pans.

2. In a bowl, combine almond flour, baking powder, xylitol, and salt.

3. In another bowl, whisk coconut cream, butter, water and vanilla to combine.

4. Add the coconut cream mixture to the almond flour mixture. Stir until well combined. Fold in chocolate chips.

5. Divide batter (it will be somewhat thick) in pan compartments, using about 1 rounded tablespoon per muffin. Bake 15-20 minutes, or until lightly browned on top and toothpick inserted in center comes out clean.

6. Cool muffins in pans for 2 minutes, then turn out onto wire racks to cool completely.

OLD FASHIONED BREAD PUDDING

Total Time: 1hr 40 min
Prep: 40 min
Cook: 1hr

8 Servings
1 Whole-Food Fat Per Serving

Ingredients

- 1/2 cup Xylitol
- 1 cup Coconut Cream
- 1 cup Tap Water

- 6 large Eggs (Whole)
- 1 tsp Vanilla Extract
- 1 tsp Cinnamon
- 8 servings SANE Bread

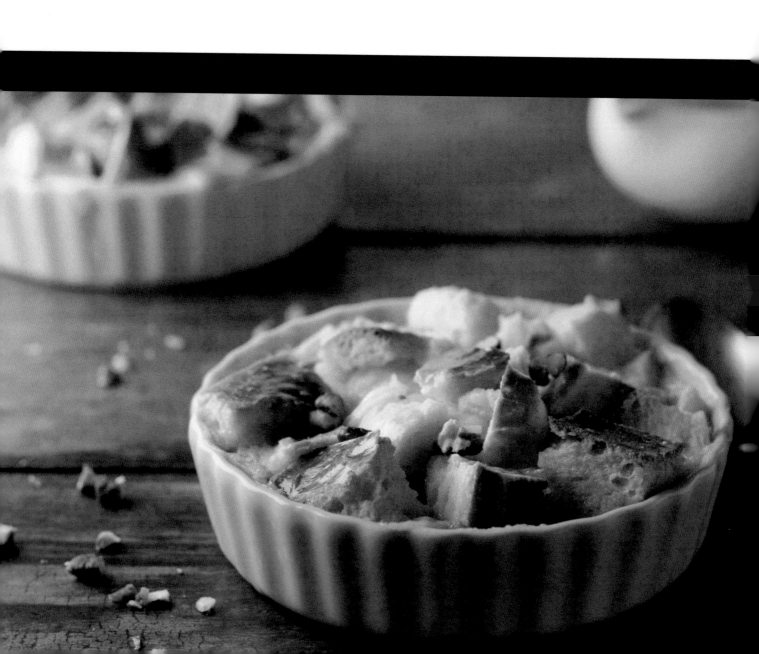

Directions

1. Preheat oven to 350°F. Generously butter a 9×9 -inch baking pan; set aside.

2. In a large bowl, whisk together eggs and xylitol.

3. In a medium saucepan over medium heat, bring coconut cream, water, vanilla and cinnamon to a boil. Slowly whisk hot cream mixture into egg mixture. Add SANE Bread and toss well. Let stand 10 minutes, turning occasionally with a rubber spatula.

4. Transfer pudding mixture into to prepared pan. Place pan in a larger roasting pan, fill the outer pan with enough hot water to come half way up the sides of the pudding pan.

5. Bake for until set, about 55 minutes. Let cool for 15 minutes before cutting. Serve warm or chilled. Makes 6 servings.

PEAR TART

Total Time: 1hr 10 min
Prep: 50 min
Cook: 20 min

6 Servings
3 Whole-Food Fats Per Serving

Ingredients

- 3/4 cup Almond Flour
- 9 tbsps Xylitol
- 4 tbsps Unsalted Butter
- 11 ozs Coconut Cream
- 2 small (approx 3 per lb) Pear
- 1 fl oz (no ice) Brandy
- 1/2 tsp Pure Almond Extract
- 1/2 tsp Ginger (Ground)
- 2 tbsps Sugar Free Apricot Preserves
- 1 large Egg (Whole)
- 2 tsps Tap Water
- 1 oz Almonds

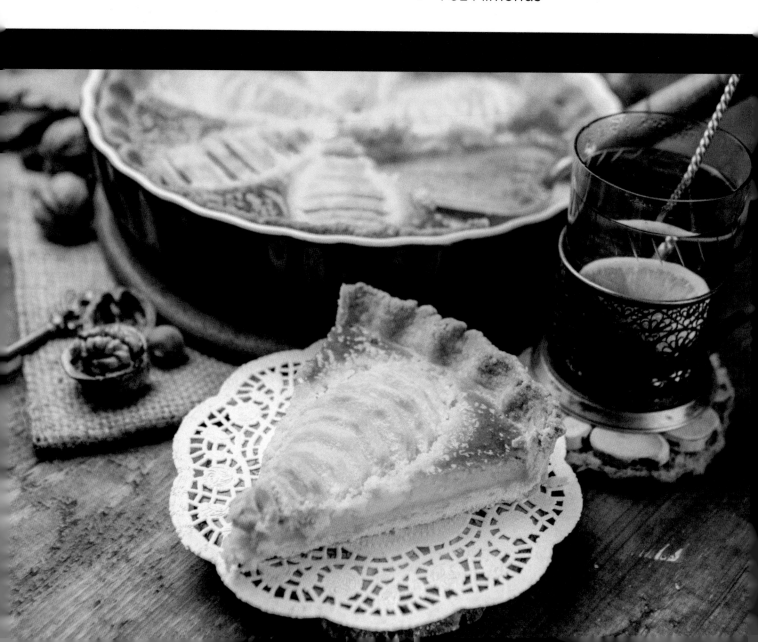

Directions

1. Preheat oven to 350°F.

2. For crust: In a food processor, pulse almond flour and 2 tablespoons xylitol to combine, about 10 seconds. Add butter and pulse until mixture resembles a coarse meal, about 30 seconds.

3. Add 3 ounces coconut cream and pulse until the dough starts to come together, about 30 more seconds. Put dough on the bottom and up the sides of an ungreased 10 tart pan.

4. Prick dough about 15 times with a fork and chill in freezer while preparing filling.

5. For filling: In a small bowl, toss pear slices with 1 tablespoon of the xylitol, Cognac, 1/4 teaspoon of the almond extract and ginger until evenly distributed. Set aside.

6. In a large bowl with an electric mixer on high speed, beat 8 ounces coconut cream at room temperature and 1/3 cup xylitol until soft and creamy, about 3 minutes. Add egg and remaining 1/4 teaspoon almond extract; beat until smooth, 1 minute more (scrape down sides of bowl as necessary).

7. Pour coconut cream mixture into chilled tart shell. Arrange pears on top of coconut cream mixture in slightly overlapping concentric circles. If there is liquid left from the pears, pour it evenly over the tart.

8. Bake for 30 minutes. Remove from oven and place on a wire rack to cool. Melt jam with water over medium heat. Brush over hot tart and sprinkle with almonds. Let tart cool completely before serving.

PINEAPPLE-MANGO LAYER CAKE

Total Time: 1hr 10 min
Prep: 50 min
Cook: 20 min

8 Servings
1 Whole-Food Fat Per Serving

Ingredients

- 1/2 fruit Pineapple
- 1/2 cup sliced Mangos
- 1 cup Whole Grain Almond Flour
- 1 tsp Baking Powder
- 1/4 tsp Salt
- 6 large Eggs (Whole)
- 2 tsps Pure Almond Extract
- 1/4 cup Unsalted Butter
- 1/2 cup Coconut Cream
- 13 tbsp Xylitol

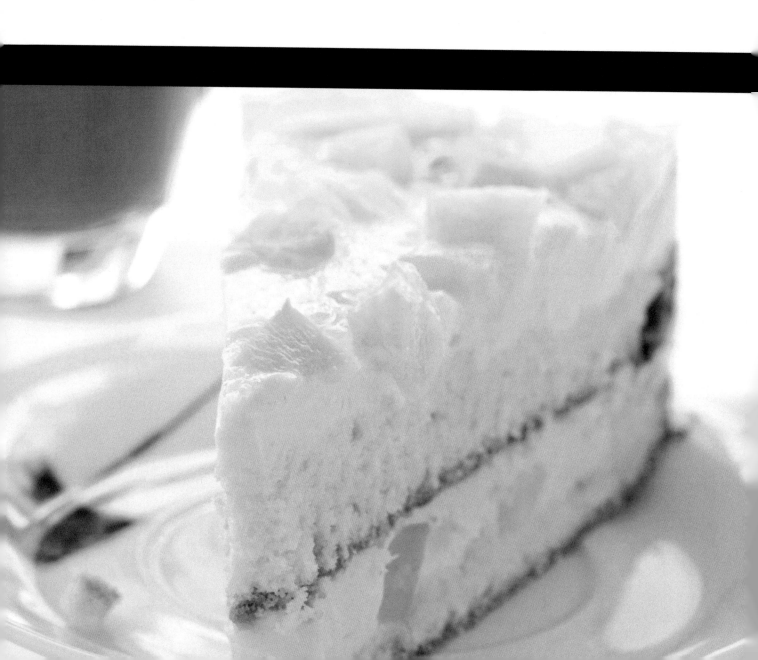

Directions

1. For cake: Preheat oven to 350°F. Line two 8-inch-round cake pans with parchment paper, grease and dust with almond flour.

2. Core the pineapple (cut off green outsides) and peel the mango. Dice all or leave about half of the pineapple in half-rings and half of the mango in slices for a decorative top; set aside.

3. In a medium bowl, whisk together almond flour, baking powder and salt. Separate the egg yolks from the whites. Set yolks aside.

4. In a large bowl with an electric mixer on medium speed, beat whites until frothy, about 3 minutes. Slowly add 3/4 cup (12 Tbsp) xylitol and continue beating until stiff, but not dry, peaks form, about 4 minutes.

5. In a small bowl, whisk together yolks, almond extract and melted butter. Slowly pour yolk mixture into the beaten egg whites and continue mixing on medium speed until yolks are combined, about 1 minute.

6. In three additions, gently fold the dry ingredients into the egg white mixture using a rubber spatula.

7. Divide batter in prepared pans; smooth tops.

8. Bake until a toothpick inserted in centers comes out clean, about 20 minutes.

9. Cool on wire rack for 5 minutes, then turn out to cool completely.

10. To assemble: In a small bowl with an electric mixer on medium, whip coconut cream with 1 tablespoon xylitol until soft peaks form, about 3 minutes.

11. Place one cake layer on a serving plate.

12. Spread half the coconut cream over cake and place diced pineapple and mango pieces all around.

13. Place second layer over coconut cream. Top with remaining coconut cream and decorate top with pieces or sliced pineapple and mango.

14. For a decorative top: Starting at the edge of the cake, arrange fruit in concentric circles, alternating pineapple and mango slices.

15. Cut into 8 servings.

Get Everything You Need To Burn Fat and Prepare Delicious Meals at the SANE Store

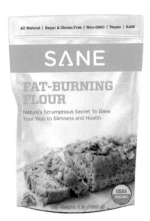

Fat-Burning Flour

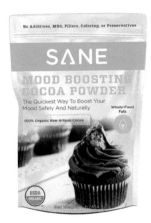

Mood-Boosting Chocolate Powder

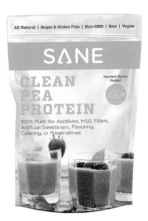

Clean Pea Protein

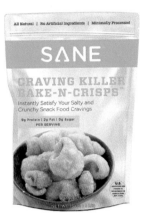

Craving Killer Bake-N-Crisps

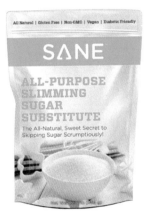

Slimming Sugar Substitute

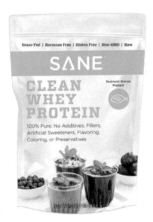

Clean Whey Protein

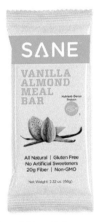

Vanilla Almond Meal Bars

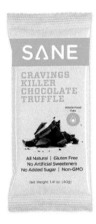

Craving Killer Chocolate Truffle

No Added Sugar

100% Natural

Gluten Free

No GMO's

No Dairy

No Soy

SANE™

Find all of these EXCLUSIVE tools, plus over 100 other fat-burning SANE products to help you and your family look and feel your best!

Visit Today: Store.SANESolution.com

PIE CRUST

Total Time: 30 min
Prep: 5 min
Cook: 25 min

1 Pie Crust
1 Whole-Food Fat Per Serving

Ingredients

- 6 tbsp Coconut Flour
- 1/4 cup Extra Virgin Coconut oil
- 3 eggs
- 1 tsp SANE honey
- 1 tsp baking powder
- 1/4 tsp sea salt

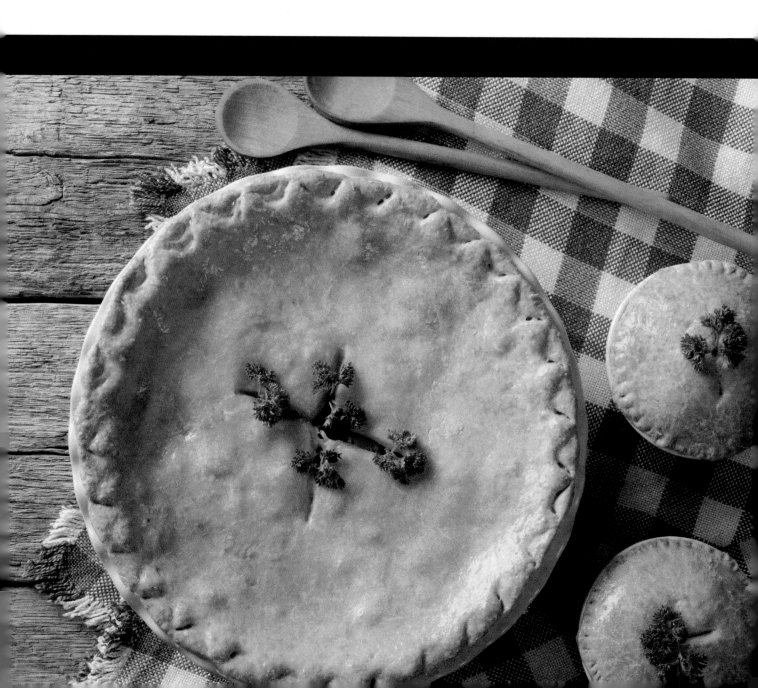

Directions

1. Preheat oven to 350 degrees F

2. Line a baking sheet with parchment paper

3. Mix together the wet ingredients in one bowl and the dry ingredients in another

4. Combine the wet and dry ingredients

5. Roll batter onto parchment paper until about 1/2 – 3/4 in thick

6. Bake for 20 minutes

PROSCIUTTO PEACH BITES

Total Time: 10 min   8 Servings
Prep: 10 min   1 Whole-Food Fat Per Serving
Cook: 0 min   1 Low-Fructose Fruits Per Serving

Ingredients

- 1 medium Peach
- 2 TBSP Coconut Cream
- 1 tsp Cinnamon

- 1/4 cup whole Almonds
- 6 leaves Basil
- 6 thin slices Prosciutto

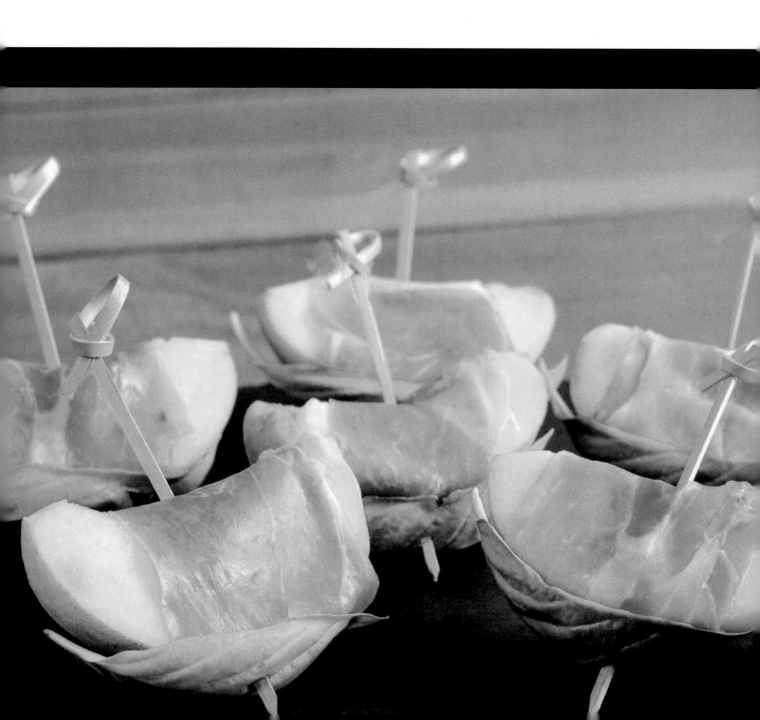

Directions

1. Preheat oven to 350°F. Toast nuts in a single layer for 10 minutes. Cool and then coarsely chop. Set aside. Slice the peach into 6 wedges and set aside.

2. In a small bowl combine the coconut cream with 1 teaspoon ground cinnamon and a pinch of stevia (optional). Add the nuts, blend to combine.

3. Lay out a single slice of prosciutto, place 1 tablespoon cheese mixture on top of peach wedge and top with a basil leaf, place the wedge at one end of the prosciutto and roll-it-up. Repeat with remaining ingredients.

PUMPKIN BACON & CHIVE BISCUITS

Total Time: 35 min
Prep: 5 min
Cook: 30 min

12 Servings
1 Whole-Food Fat Per Serving

Ingredients

- 3-4 strips of bacon
- 1/2 cup plus 2 teaspoons coconut flour
- 3/4 teaspoon baking soda
- 1/4 teaspoon salt
- 1/2 Cup Xylitol

- 1 tablespoon apple cider vinegar
- 1/2 cup pumpkin puree
- 3 large eggs
- 1/4 cup finely chopped chives or green onions

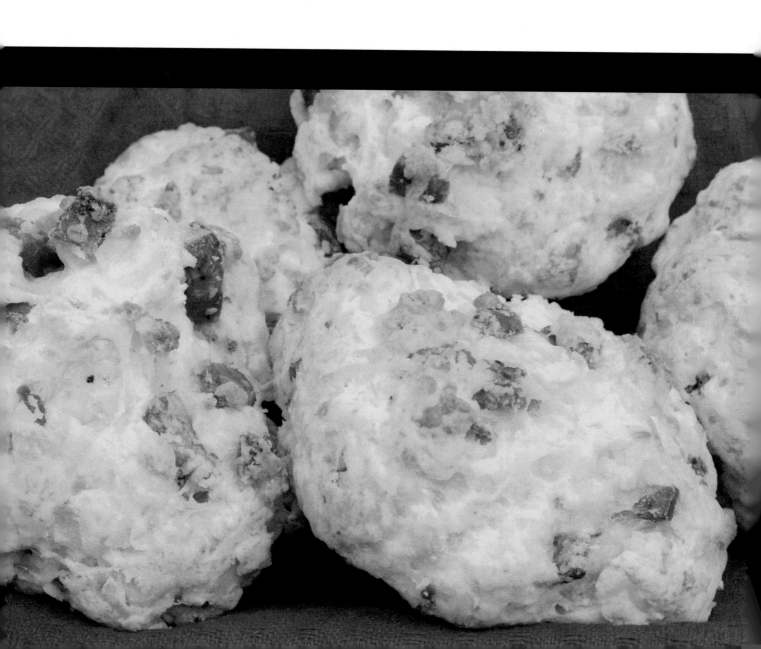

Directions

1. Preheat oven to 350F/176C, and line a large baking sheet with parchment paper.

2. Preheat a skillet over medium heat and cook the bacon until crispy. Remove bacon from the pan and leave to cool on a wire rack or paper towels. Once cool, break or cut into small pieces. Pour the bacon fat into a liquid measuring cup.

3. In a large bowl, whisk together the coconut flour, baking soda, Xylitol and salt. Set aside.

4. In another bowl, whisk together the fat, vinegar, pumpkin purée and eggs until well combined. Pour this liquid mixture into the flour mixture, and whisk till smooth.

5. Fold the bacon and chive pieces into the batter.

6. Use a 1/4 cup measuring cup or mechanical ice cream scoop to drop mounds of batter on to the baking sheet. Spacing them about 2 inches apart. Smooth and shape as needed.

7. Bake for 18-20 min or until golden around the edges. Times will vary from oven to oven and thickness of the biscuit.

8. Allow biscuits to cool for at least 5 minutes on the baking sheet before transferring from the pan. Biscuits will be fragile while hot.

9. Makes 6-7 biscuits depending on how you measure. Can be stored in an airtight container, up to one day in the fridge. After that they start to dry out.

PUMPKIN CHEESECAKE

Total Time: 4hr 45 min
Prep: 4hr
Cook: 45 min

10 Servings
2 Whole-Food Fats Per Serving

Ingredients

- 24 ozs Coconut Cheese
- 15 ozs Pumpkin (Without Salt, Canned)
- 2/3 cup Xylitol

- 1/2 tsp Vanilla Extract
- 1/2 tsp Cinnamon
- 1/4 tsp Ginger (Ground)
- 3 large Eggs (Whole)

Directions

1. Heat oven to 325°F. Spray an 8×3-inch deep cake pan with coconut oil cooking spray. Line bottom with a round of parchment or wax paper; spray paper; set aside.

2. In a large bowl, with an electric mixer on medium, beat coconut cream until smooth. Add pumpkin purée, xylitol, vanilla, cinnamon and ginger; beat until smooth.

3. Beat in eggs one at a time, just until combined. Pour batter into prepared pan. Place cake pan in a deep roasting pan and carefully pour in enough boiling water into roasting pan to reach halfway up sides of cake pan. Bake 42-45 minutes, until cake is just set in center. Turn off oven, open door and let stand in oven 15 minutes. Remove cake pan from water bath and transfer to a wire rack; cool completely. Run a knife around edge of cake, cover and refrigerate until chilled (4 hours or overnight).

4. To remove cake from pan, dip bottom of pan into hot water for just a few seconds to loosen. Place serving platter over top and invert. Remove pan and peel off paper. Garnish with mint and pecans, if desired.

PUMPKIN DONUT SANDWICHES

Total Time: 20 min
Prep: 10 min
Cook: 10 min

8 mini donuts
2 Whole-Food Fats Per Serving

Ingredients

For the donuts:
- 6 dried medjool dates, pitted
- 1/2 cup pumpkin puree
- 1/4 cup extra virgin coconut oil, melted
- 4 eggs
- 3 tablespoons coconut flour
- 1/2 tablespoon cinnamon
- 1/4 teaspoon nutmeg
- 1/8 teaspoon ground cloves
- 1/8 teaspoon ground ginger
- 1/2 teaspoon baking powder
- pinch of salt

For the cream:
- 1 (14 ounce) can of coconut cream
- 1 tablespoon maple syrup
- 1/4 teaspoon cinnamon

For the chocolate:
- 1 cup 100% Chocolate Chips, melted
- 3 tablespoons coconut milk/water

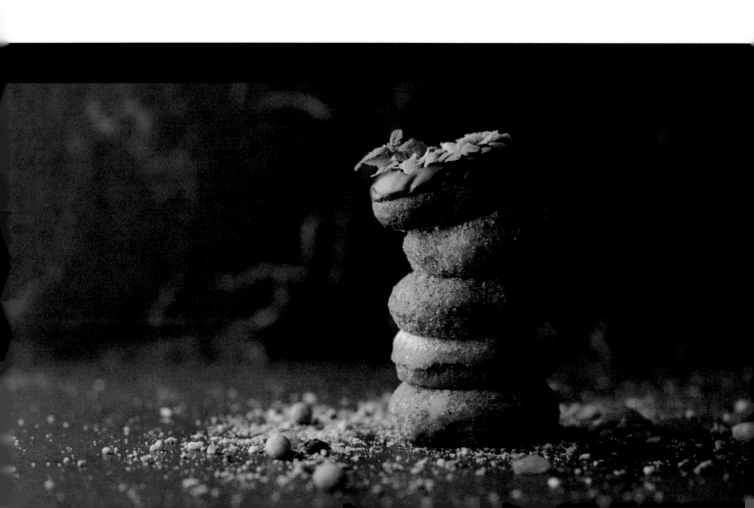

Directions

1. Place dried dates in a food processor and pulse to break down.

2. Add pumpkin puree, melted extra virgin coconut oil, and eggs to the food processor and puree until smooth.

3. Add coconut flour, cinnamon, nutmeg, ground cloves, ginger, baking powder, and a pinch of salt and puree once more.

4. To make the donuts easy to pour and keep them a round shape, place donut puree into a plastic bag or pastry bag, cut the end off of the plastic bag so you can squeeze to mixture in a circle in the donut maker.

5. If you are using a donut pan for the oven, preheat oven to 350 degrees.

6. Heat up a mini donut maker, grease the donut maker maker or pan, and use the bag to squeeze about 2 tablespoons of the mixture into each donut round.

7. In a mini donut maker, cook for 5-7 minutes. Times will vary with the different donut maker.

8. If you are using a donut pan, cook for 20-25 minutes.

9. Remove donuts once cooked through and let cool on a wire rack.

10. Once cooled, place in refrigerator for about 10 minutes. (the donuts will be easier to work with once they are a bit harder).

11. While the donuts cool, in a bowl, remove the coconut cream that sits on top of the coconut water (keep the coconut water for later) and whip together the coconut cream with a fork or whisk.

12. Then add maple syrup and cinnamon and mix well. Place cream in a piping bag or plastic bag and then cut off the end.

13. In a bowl, melt chocolate chips and coconut milk/water that was left behind from the coconut cream via a double boiler or in a microwave.

14. Cut the donuts in half, carefully. On the bottom donut, pipe on the cream around the donut then place the top donut half on top of the cream.

15. Then finish the donuts off by dipping them halfway into the melted chocolate.

16. Place donuts on a parchment lined baking sheet and into the freezer to harden the chocolate.

17. Once chocolate has hardened, eat up!

18. Yields 8 mini donuts.

PUMPKIN MUFFINS

Total Time: 35 min
Prep: 10 min
Cook: 25 min

10 muffins
1 Whole-Food Fat Per Serving

Ingredients

- 1/2 cup coconut flour
- 4 eggs
- 1/4 cup extra virgin coconut oil
- 6 tbsps pumpkin purée (or squash or carrot purée)
- 2 tbsps SANE honey

- 1 tsp cinnamon or pumpkin pie spice
- 1/4 tsp ground ginger
- 1 tsp vanilla extract
- 1 tsp apple cider vinegar
- 1/4 tsp baking soda

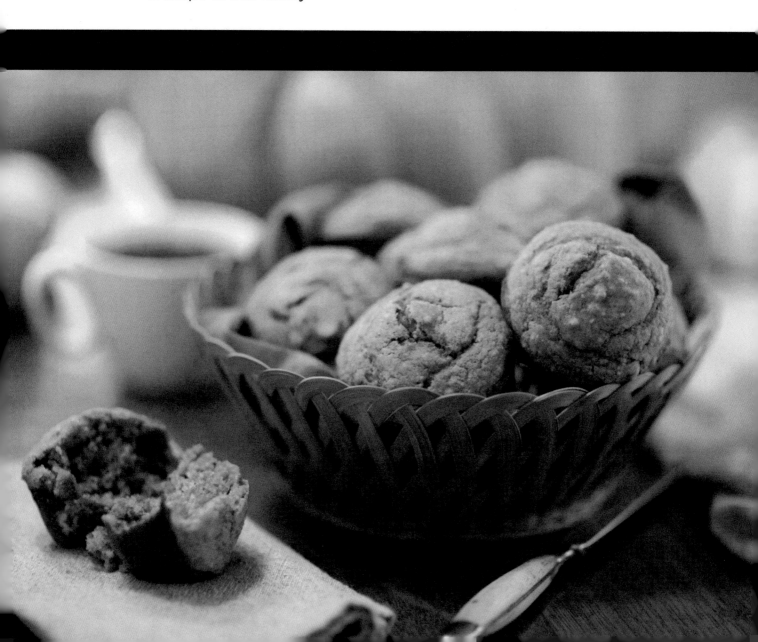

Directions

1. Preheat the oven to 350 degrees and line 10 muffin cups with liners.

2. Stir together the coconut flour and eggs until a smooth paste forms. Stir in the butter/lard, then the pumpkin pureé and honey. Then mix in the spices, cider vinegar and baking soda.

3. Divide between prepared muffin pan. Bake for about 25-30 minutes, until golden and the top springs back when lightly pressed.

Pumpkin Pie Topped with Meringue and Toasted Nuts

Total Time: 1hr 15 min
Prep: 15 min
Cook: 1hr

8 Servings
3 Whole-Food Fats Per Serving

Ingredients

- 1/3 cup Almond Flour
- 1 cup chopped Pecan Nuts
- 1 1/4 cup Xylitol
- 6 tbsps Unsalted Butter
- 1 fl oz Tap Water
- 15 ozs Pumpkin (Without Salt, Canned)
- 1 tsp Cinnamon
- 3/4 tsp Ginger (Ground)
- 1/4 tsp Cloves (Ground)
- 1/4 tsp Salt
- 2 large Eggs (Whole)
- 3 large Egg Whites
- 1 1/2 cups Coconut Cream
- 2 servings All Purpose SANE Baking Mix

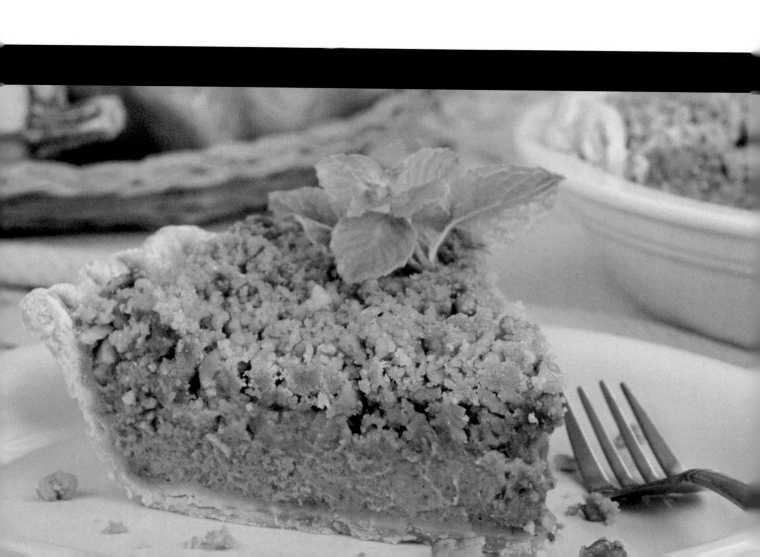

Directions

1. Heat oven to 425ºF.

2. In a large bowl whisk together almond flour, 2/3 cup All Purpose SANE Baking Mix, pecans (chop finely) and 1/4 cup xylitol. Cut in butter with a pastry blender or two knives until butter pieces are about the size of peas. Add the ice water; stir to combine.

3. Transfer crust mixture to a 9-inch pie plate. Press along bottom and sides of pie plate to form a crust. Place in freezer to harden, about 15 minutes.

4. Cover crust with aluminum foil and bake 15 minutes; remove from oven and take off foil. Reduce oven to 375ºF.

5. In a bowl, whisk pumpkin purée, 3/4 cup xylitol, ground cinnamon, ginger, cloves, and salt to combine. Mix in eggs, one at a time. Add coconut cream and mix well.

6. Pour filling into partially baked pie crust. Cover crust edge with aluminum foil. Bake 40 minutes, or until filling is set but still a little jiggly in the middle. Cool on a wire rack while you make the meringue but turn the oven down to 350°F..

For meringue and toasted nut topping:

1. Whip egg whites and coconut cream with an electric beater until frothy.

2. Slowly add 1/4 cup xylitol until fully incorporated then whip at high speed until stiff glossy peaks form.

3. Top pie with meringue and then sprinkle the 1/2 cup finely chopped nuts on top.

4. Place in the oven and continue to bake for 15-20 minutes until the nuts are toasted and browned.

5. Cool on a wire rack until ready to serve.

6. The pie may be made up to 3 days prior to serving, but do not add the meringue until you are ready to serve. Be sure the pie has warmed to room temperature if previously chilled before adding and cooking the meringue and nuts (otherwise your pie plate may crack with the sudden change in temperature). The meringue topping will not keep more than a day once made.

PUMPKIN POTS

Total Time: 48 min
Prep: 10 min
Cook: 38 min

6 Servings
1 Whole-Food Fat Per Serving

Ingredients

- 2 large Eggs (Whole)
- 2 large Egg Yolks
- 14 oz Coconut Cream
- 1 tsp Vanilla Extract
- 15 ozs Pumpkin (Without Salt, Canned)
- 1/4 cup Xylitol

- 1 pinch Stevia
- 1/4 cup Sugar Free Maple Flavored Syrup
- 1 tsp Ginger (Ground)
- 1 tsp Cinnamon
- 1/4 tsp Nutmeg (Ground)
- 3/4 tsp Salt

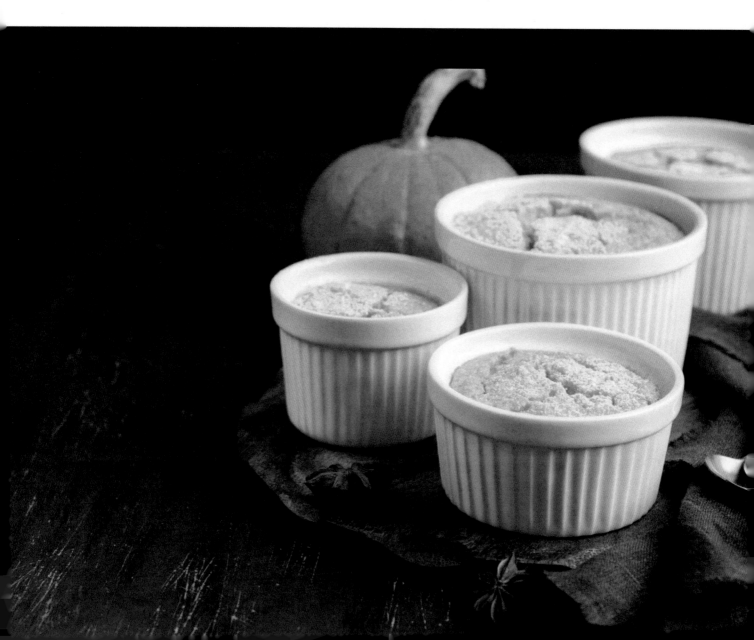

Directions

1. Preheat oven to 400°F. Lightly grease 6 ramekins; set aside. You will also need a pan big enough to accommodate all the ramekins and deep enough to hold 1-inch of water without spilling into the ramekins.

2. Whisk the whole eggs and yolks with the coconut milk and vanilla in a medium bowl. Set aside.

3. In a medium sauce pot combine the pumpkin, xylitol, maple syrup, ginger, ground cinnamon, nutmeg and salt. Cook over medium-high heat until reduced slightly, fragrant and shiny; about 15 minutes stirring often to prevent burning on the bottom of the pan. Remove from heat and quickly whisk in the egg mixture.

4. Divide mixture into 6 ramekins (do not overfill) and place in a deep sided pan. Fill the pan with hot water until it reaches about 1-inch up the side of the ramekins. Place in oven and bake for 10 minutes at 400°F then reduce heat to 300°F and cook an additional 25-30 minutes or until the centers jiggle only slightly in the center.

5. Remove from oven and allow to sit in the water bath to cool to room temperature. These are wonderful eaten warm about 20 minutes after baking or cold after being refrigerated for at least 3 hours or up to 2 days. Store leftovers in the refrigerator covered with plastic wrap and eat within 1 week.

6. Top with a dollop of coconut cream just before serving if desired.

Pumpkin Raisin Cookies

Total Time: 35 min
Prep: 5 min
Cook: 30 min

15 cookies
1 Whole-Food Fat Per Serving

Ingredients

For the cookies:
- 2/3 cup coconut flour
- 6 tbsps extra virgin coconut oil
- 2 eggs
- 1/2 cup pumpkin puree
- 1/4 cup SANE honey
- 1/2 tsp baking soda
- 1/2 tsp raw apple cider vinegar
- Pinch of unrefined salt

- 1/2 tsp ground cinnamon
- Pinch of freshly grated nutmeg
- 1/2 tsp vanilla extract
- 1/2 cup organic raisins

For the frosting:
- 1/4 cup coconut cream
- 1/4 cup SANE honey
- 2 tsp coconut milk or milk of choice
- 1/2 tsp vanilla extract

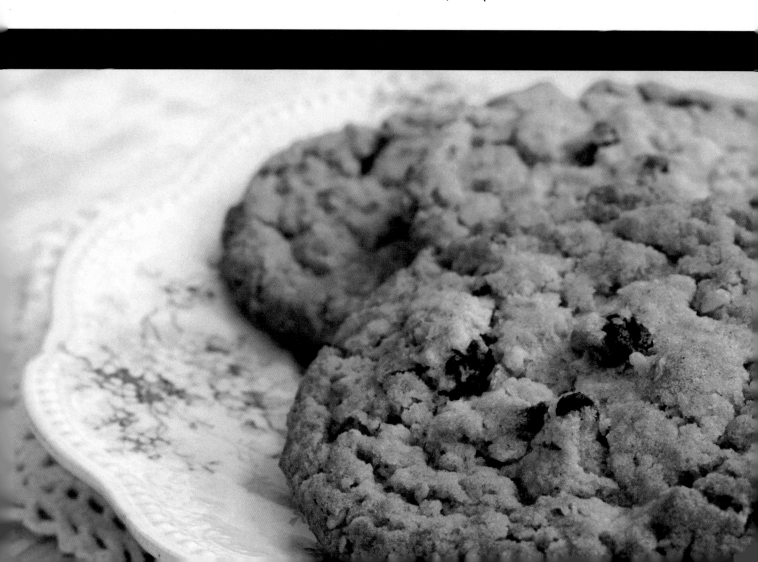

Directions

1. Preheat the oven to 350. To measure the coconut flour, fluff flour with a fork then scoop the measuring cup and level. Don't pack the flour, or the cookies will be too heavy.

2. Have all ingredients at room temperature and then stir together until well combined. If ingredients are not at room temperature, the batter will not combine because the coconut oil will clump. You can melt the coconut oil to help it mix together well.

3. Flatten balls of dough on a parchment paper lined baking sheet. I recommend making them smaller than the cookies in the picture – the bigger the cookies, the more fragile. I suggest using 1 tbs. of dough per cookie and just flattening it slightly.

4. Bake for 18-20 minutes, until golden around the edges. Cool cookies completely before frosting.

5. To make the frosting, have the ingredients at room temperature. Stir together until creamy. You may need to add another teaspoon or more of coconut milk for a spreadable frosting. Frost cookies before serving. Cookies and frosting should be stored separately. These cookies freeze relatively well.

PUMPKIN-SPICE BROWNIES

Total Time: 40 min
Prep: 10 min
Cook: 30 min

16 Servings
1 Whole-Food Fat Per Serving

Ingredients

- 2 ozs Unsweetened Baking Chocolate Squares
- 1/2 cup Unsalted Butter
- 1 cup Erythritol
- 1 tbsp SANE Cocoa Powder
- 2 tsps Vanilla Extract
- 4 large Eggs (Whole)

- 4 tbsps Almond Flour
- 1/4 tsp Baking Soda
- 1/4 tsp Salt
- 1/2 tsp Cinnamon
- 8 ozs Coconut Cream
- 2/3 cup Pumpkin (Without Salt, Canned)
- 1 1/2 tsps Pumpkin Pie Spice

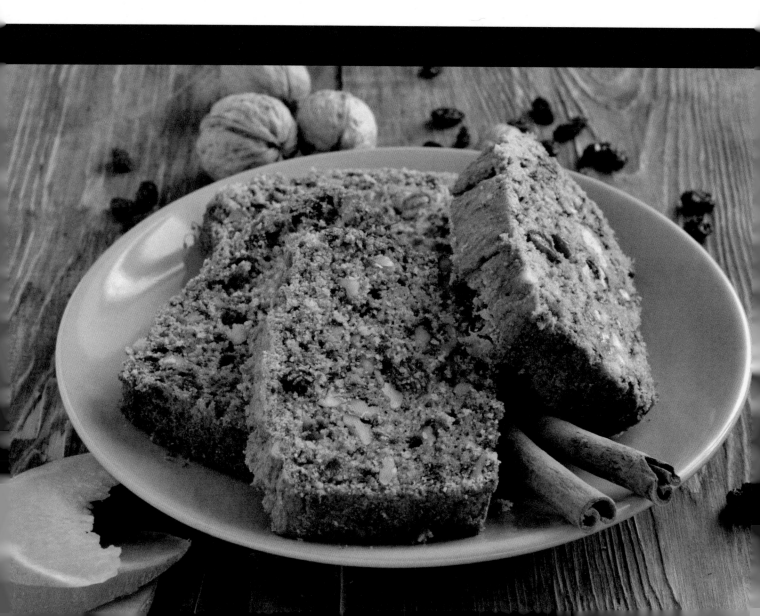

Directions

1. Preheat an oven to 350°F. Grease an 8×8-inch pan.

2. Melt the butter and chocolate in a small bowl at 30 second intervals in the microwave until melted.

3. Thoroughly blend the chocolate and butter together then add in SANE Cocoa Powder and 1/2 cup erythritol and continue to blend until smooth.

4. Add 1 teaspoon vanilla and 3 eggs; whisk until incorporated.

5. Combine the almond flour, baking soda, salt and cinnamon in a small bowl. Add to the chocolate mixture and stir until thickened. Set the brownie mixture aside.

6. Using a hand blender cream the coconut cream with the rest of erythritol in a small bowl.

7. Add 1 egg, pumpkin purée, pumpkin spice blend and 1 teaspoon vanilla; beat until smooth.

8. Spread 2/3 of the brownie mixture into the prepared pan. Then pour the coconut cream mixture over the top.

9. Drop the remaining 1/3 of the brownie batter by spoonfuls over the coconut cream mixture and then take a knife and gently swirl the layers together.

10. Bake for 30 minutes until a tooth pick inserted in the center comes out clean.

11. Allow to cool before cutting. Best served at room temperature but keep refrigerated in an airtight container for up to 1 week.

RASPBERRY PARFAIT

Total Time: 5 min
Prep: 5 min
Cook: 0 min

2 Servings
4 Whole-Food Fats Per Serving

Ingredients

- 1/2 cup Cocunut Cream
- 4 ozs Mascarpone

- 4 TBSP Xylitol
- 1/2 cup Raspberries

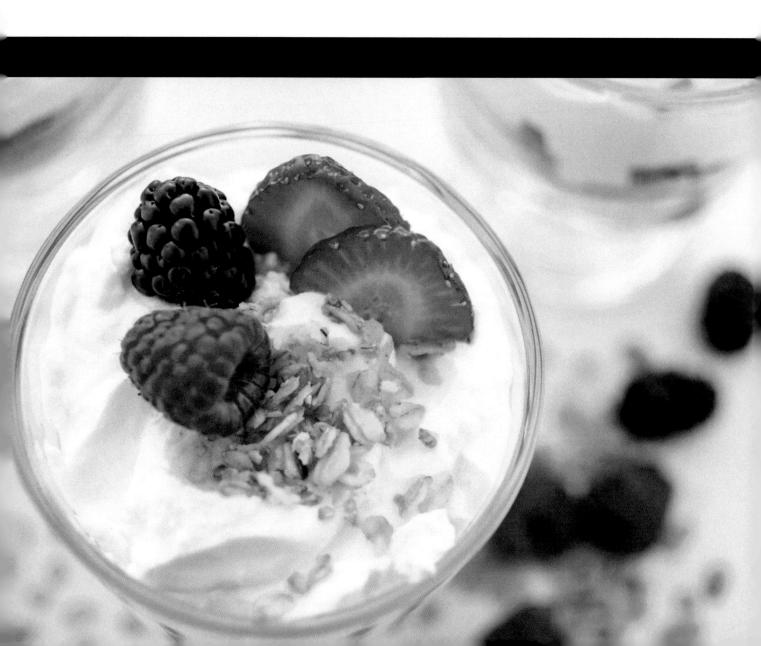

Directions

1. Beat 1/2 cup coconut cream until soft peaks form.

2. Add 4 oz mascarpone and xylitol. Beat just until smooth.

3. Using 1/2 cup raspberries, layer with the dairy mixture in 2 parfait glasses.

SANE Almond Cookies

Total Time: 20 min
Prep: 10 min
Cook: 10 min

24 Servings
1 Whole-Food Fat Per Serving

Ingredients

- 1/2 cup Blanched & Slivered Almonds
- 3/4 cup Almond Flour
- 3 tsps Baking Powder
- 3/4 cup Xylitol

- 1 large Egg (Whole)
- 1 large Egg Yolk
- 2 tsps Vanilla Extract
- 1/4 cup Unsalted Butter

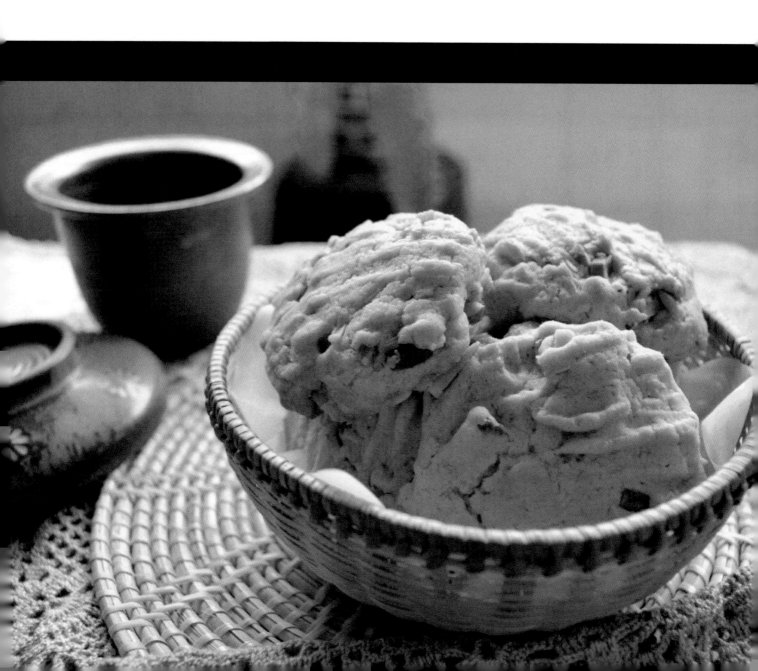

Directions

1. Preheat oven to 375°F. In a food processor, finely grind the almonds with the almond flour, baking powder, and xylitol.

2. In a separate bowl, with an electric mixer on medium, beat whole egg and egg yolk, vanilla and butter until well incorporated (mixture will not attain a smooth consistency). With a rubber spatula, fold in soy mixture just until combined.

3. Form dough into 24 small balls; arrange on an ungreased baking sheet. Lightly flatten them with a fork to silver dollar size.

4. Bake 8 to 10 minutes, until set. Cool on baking sheets before transferring to a wire rack.

SANE Caramel Sauce

Total Time: 25 min
Prep: 5 min
Cook: 20 min

6 Servings
1 Whole-Food Fat Per Serving

Ingredients

- 1 can coconut milk
- 1/4 cup SANE honey
- 3/4 cup Xylitol

- 1 tbsp Extra Virgin Coconut oil
- 1 tsp vanilla extract
- 1/2 tsp sea salt

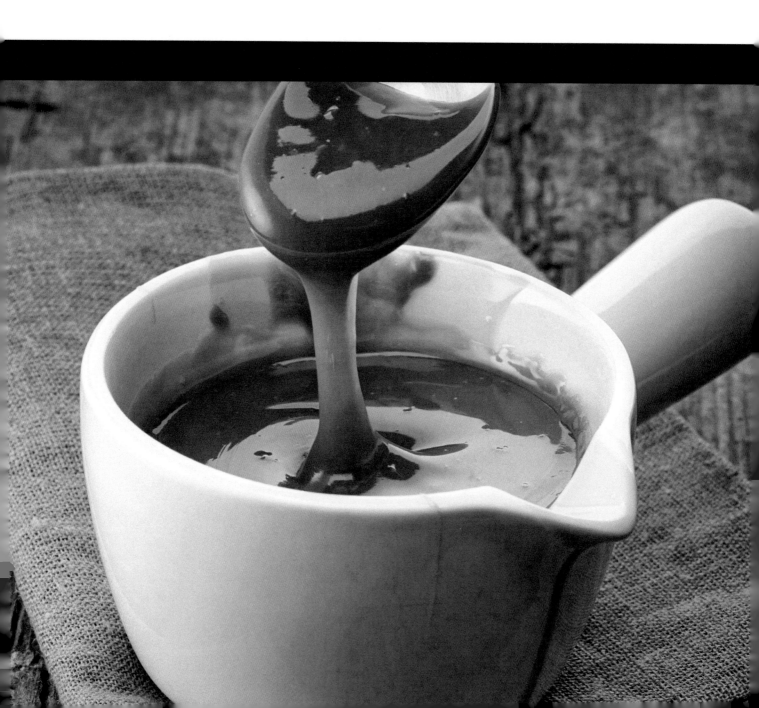

Directions

1. Place coconut milk, xylitol and SANE honey in a saucepan. Bring to a boil and then reduce the heat and allow to simmer for 15 minutes.

2. Add in extra virgin coconut oil, vanilla and sea salt and mix. Place in fridge and allow mixture to cool completely before serving.

SANE Chocolate Cake

Total Time: 13 min
Prep: 5 min
Cook: 8 min

4 Servings
2 Whole-Food Fats Per Serving

Ingredients

- 6 tbsps Unsalted Butter
- 2 ozs Baking Chocolate Squares
- 2 large Egg Yolks

- 1 tbsp Almond Flour
- 2 large Eggs (Whole)
- 1/3 cup Xylitol
- 1 tsp Vanilla Extract

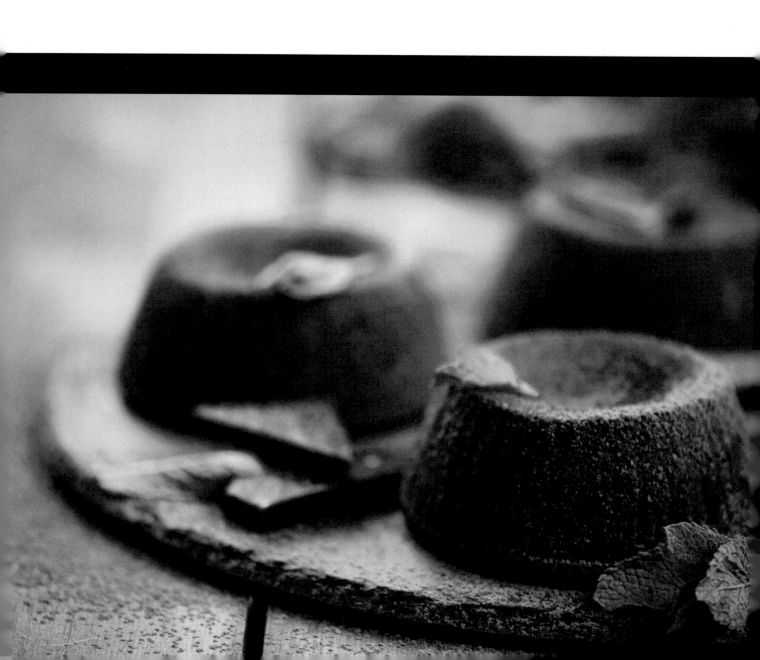

Directions

1. Preheat oven to 375°F.

2. Generously grease four 6-ounce custard cups with butter and dust with xylitol. Place cups on a baking sheet.

3. Place butter and chocolate in a double boiler over medium heat and cook until just melted, about 3 minutes (or 1 minute in a microwave on high). Remove from heat and let cool to room temperature.

4. Pour chocolate mixture into a large bowl; add almond flour and stir until just combined. Set aside.

5. In a large bowl, beat eggs, egg yolks, xylitol and vanilla with an electric mixer on high speed until almost firm peaks form, about 4 minutes.

6. In three additions, fold egg mixture into chocolate mixture.

7. Divide batter in cups. Bake 8-9 minutes until a toothpick inserted near edge comes out clean and inserted in center comes out with some batter.

8. Cool 3 minutes. Run knife around edge, turn upside down to release onto serving plates. Serve immediately. Makes 4 servings.

SANE CHOCOLATE-MINT MOUSSE

Total Time: 35 min
Prep: 35 min
Cook: 0 min

8 Servings
1 Whole-Food Fat Per Serving

Ingredients

- 1 1/2 cups Coconut Cream
- 1 1/2 oz Clean Whey Protein

- 1 1/2 oz Mood Boosting Cocoa Powder
- 1/2 teaspoon mint extract

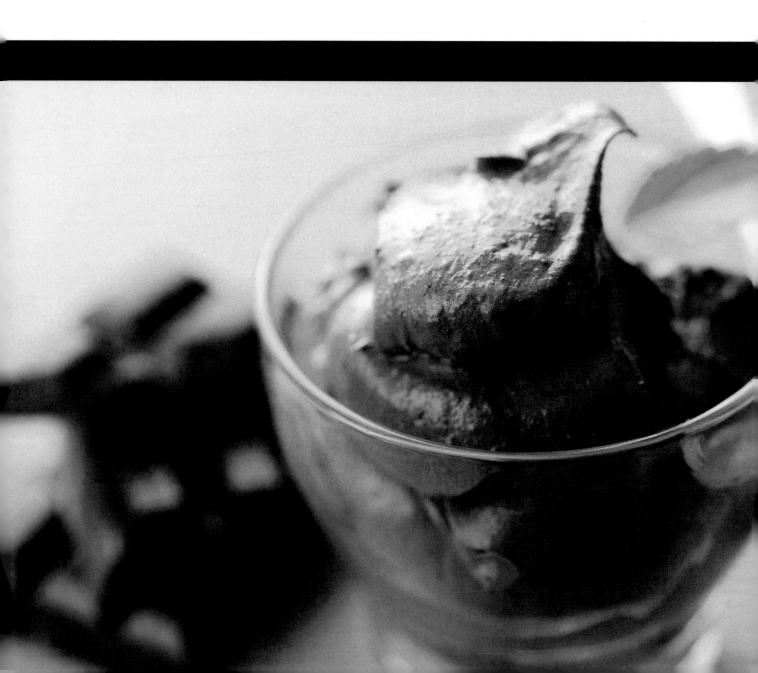

Directions

1. Beat coconut cream with an electric mixer until thickened.

2. Add SANE Clean Whey Protein, Mood Boosting Cocoa Powder, and extract; continue beating until smooth and firm.

3. Chill 30 minutes.

SANE CINNAMON PIE CRUST

Total Time: 10 min
Prep: 10 min
Cook: 0 min

8 Servings
1 Whole-Food Fat Per Serving

Ingredients

- 1/4 tsp Salt
- 1 tsp Xylitol
- 1 tsp Cinnamon

- 1/2 cup Unsalted Butter Stick
- 1 1/3 cup All Purpose SANE Baking Mix
- 2 tbsps Tap Water

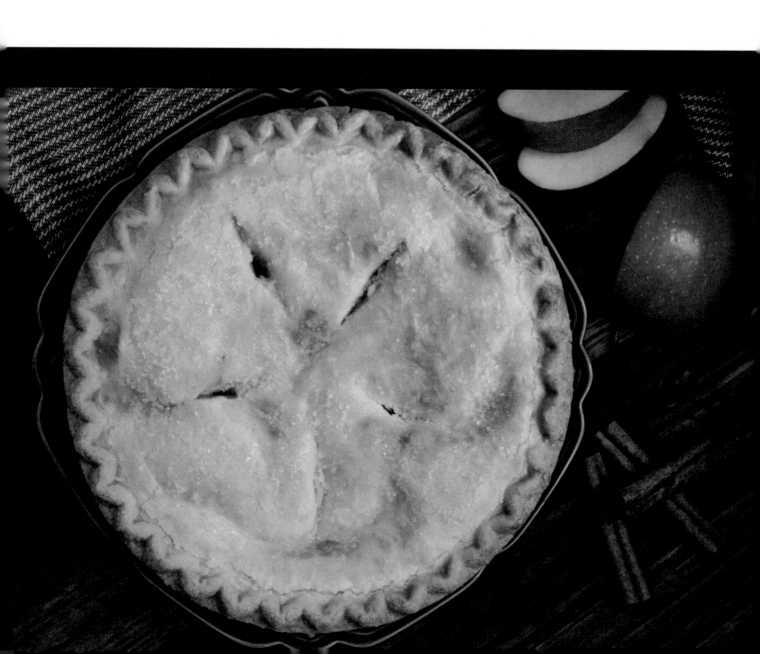

Directions

1. Pulse the All Purpose SANE Baking Mix, salt, xylitol, and cinnamon in a food processor to incorporate; add butter and pulse until mixture resembles a coarse meal, about 30 seconds. Pulse in water until dough just comes together, about 30 seconds (add up to 1 more tablespoon if necessary).

2. Transfer dough to a sheet of plastic wrap; form into a a disk about 6 inches in diameter. Wrap tightly in plastic; refrigerate until firm, about 30 minutes.

3. Roll and bake as directed in pie recipe. Makes 1 pie crust.

SANE Honey

Total Time: 5 min
Prep: 5 min
Cook: 0 min

Ingredients

- 1 ½ Cups Xylitol
- ¼ Cup Water
- ½ to 1 TSP Guar Gum

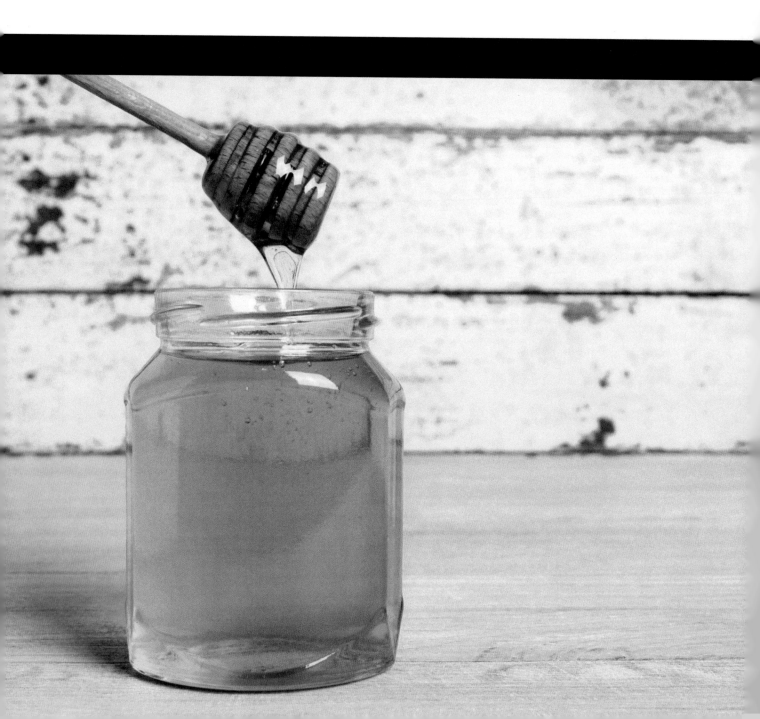

Directions

1. Place 1/2 TSP guar gum, water, and xylitol into a blender or food processor.

2. Blend completely

3. Add up to another 1/2 TSP of guar gum (1/8 TSP at a time) until you reach the desired consistency

4. Remove SANE Honey using a spatula and refrigerate for at least 20 minutes before using.

TIP: For a thinner consistency, add more water 1 TSP at a time. For a thicker consistency, add more guar gum 1/8 TSP at a time

SANE Coconut Cake

Total Time: 57 min
Prep: 20 min
Cook: 37 min

16 Servings
3 Whole-Food Fats Per Serving

Ingredients

- 2 cups Unsalted Butter
- 13 tbsps Xylitol
- 2 tsps Vanilla Extract
- 3 tsps Coconut Extract
- 6 large Eggs (Whole)
- 3/4 cups Almond Flour

- 1 tsp Baking Powder
- 1 tsp Salt
- 1 cup Coconut Milk Unsweetened
- 1 cup Dried Coconut
- 16 ozs Coconut Cream

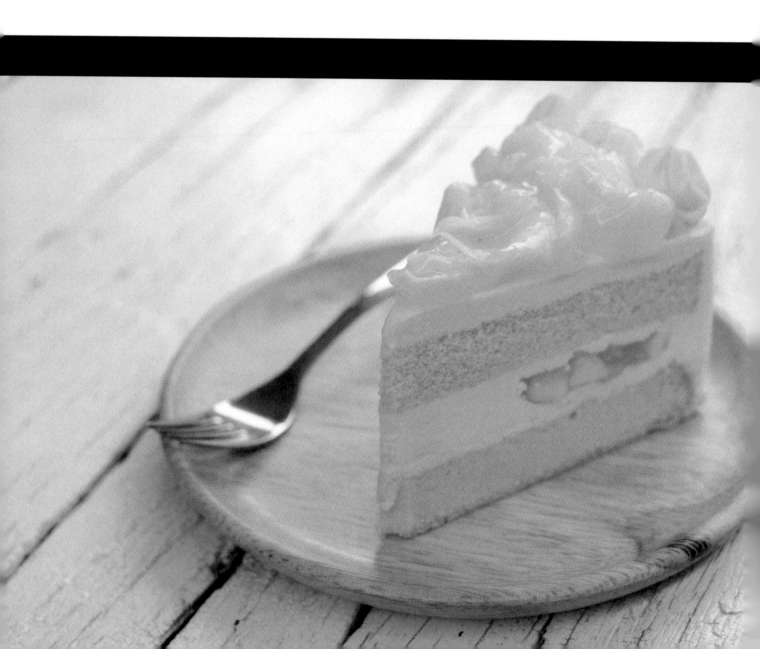

Directions

1. Preheat oven to 325°F. Prepare two 9-inch round pans with coconut oil spray, cut out parchment paper to fit into the bottom of each pan, place the paper in the pan and spray it with oil. Set aside.

2. With an electric mixer beat 1 cup butter and then the 8 tbsps of xylitol that was powdered until light and fluffy, about 3 minutes. Add the vanilla and 2 tsp coconut extract; blend to combine. Add the eggs one at a time blending after each addition; the mixture may separate a bit at this point.

3. Sift together 3/4 cup almond flour, baking powder and salt. Add to butter mixture and mix until thoroughly combined. Add in the coconut milk and 1/2 cup shredded coconut, blend until incorporated. Scoop into prepared pans and spread evenly with a spatula.

4. Bake for 35-40 minutes until cakes begin to pull away from the pans and are fully set in the center. Cool for 10 minutes in the pan, remove from pan and then cool on a rack. The cakes will be a little fragile so be careful handling them. Place cooled cakes in the refrigerator until ready to frost and serve. Frost just before serving.

5. Frosting: with an electric mixer blend the coconut cream and 1 cup butter until smooth. Add the 5 tbsps of xylitol that was powdered and 1 teaspoon coconut extract; blend until light and fluffy. Use 1/3 of the frosting to frost between the layers and the remaining to frost the top and the sides of the cake.

6. Toast the remaining 1/2 cup shredded coconut in the oven at 350°F for 5 minutes until lightly browned. Sprinkle coconut on top of the cake and along sides if desired. Refrigerate any remaining cake for up to one week.

SANE Iced Doughnuts

Total Time: 10 min
Prep: 3 min
Cook: 7 min

1 Serving
1 Nutrient-Dense Protein Per Serving

Ingredients

- 4 TBSP Clean Whey or Pea Protein
- 1 TBSP Coconut Flour
- 1 TBSP SANE Cocoa Powder
- 2 to 3 TBSP Belly-Busting Sugar Substitute for Baking (xylitol) (adjust to taste)
- 1 TSP Baking Powder
- 1/3 Cup Coconut Milk (may need an additional TBSP)
- 1 Egg
- Coconut oil

For Icing:
- 2 TBSP Clean Whey or Pea Protein
- 1 to 3 TBSP Belly-Busting Sugar Substitute for Baking (xylitol) (adjust to taste)
- 2 TBSP Non-Fat Greek Yogurt
- Pinch of salt

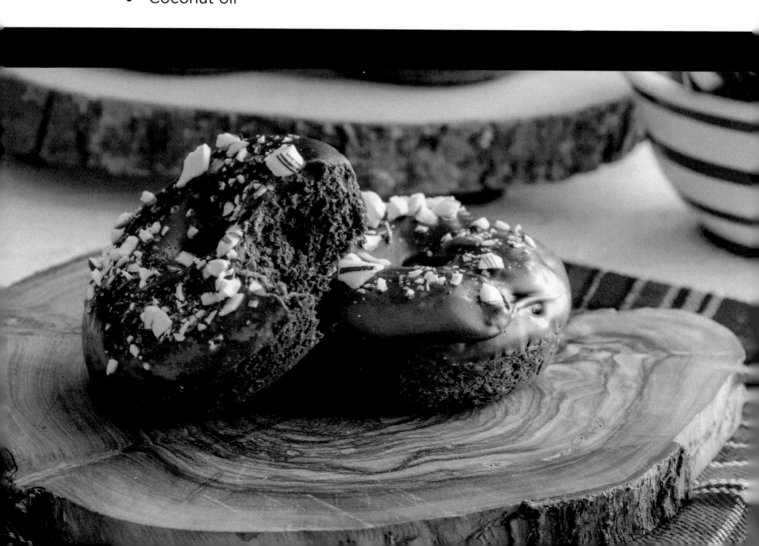

Directions

1. Mix all ingredients thoroughly in a bowl.

2. Lightly grease a donut baking dish with coconut oil

3. Place mixture evenly in baking dish

4. Bake at 350 for about 7 minutes

5. While baking, mix icing ingredients in a bowl

6. Remove donuts from oven

7. Remove donuts from baking dish and apply icing while still warm

8. (Optional) Sprinkle unsweetened shredded coconut or crushed sugar free peppermint candy over the donuts.

SANE Pie Crust 2.0

Total Time: 25 min
Prep: 10 min
Cook: 15 min

10 Servings
1 Whole-Food Fat Per Serving

Ingredients

- 1 3/4 cup almond flour
- 3 tbsp. coconut flour
- 1/2 tsp. baking powder

- 3 tbsp. Xylitol
- 1 egg white
- 1/2 tsp. vanilla extract
- 1/4 cup salted butter, melted

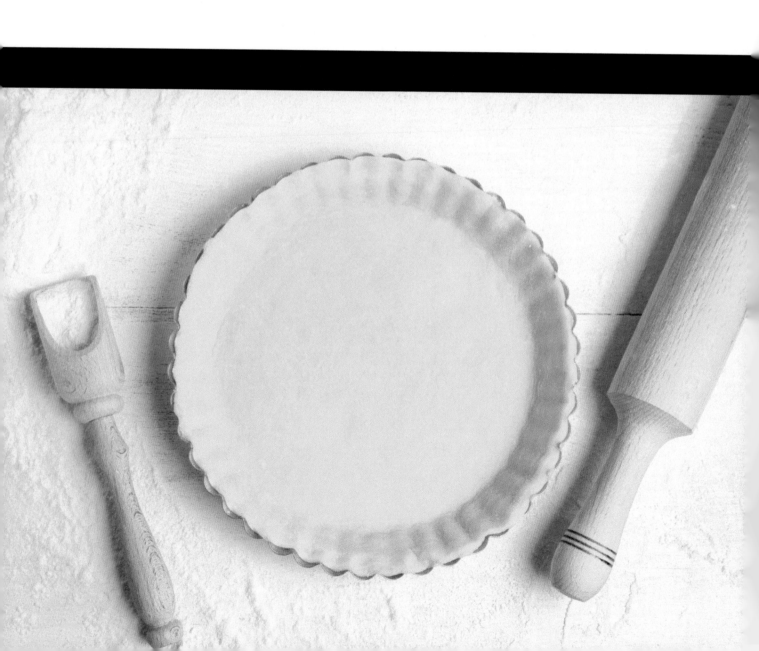

Directions

1. Preheat oven to 325 degrees F. In medium bowl, add the dry ingredients. Blend well with a whisk. Add the remaining ingredients and blend with a wooden spoon until a stiff dough forms. Taste for sweetness and adjust if needed.

2. Place dough on parchment paper and top with a piece of plastic wrap. Roll out dough with rolling pin to uniform thickness and until the dough is about 11 inches in diameter. Remove the plastic wrap and invert the pie crust into a 9 or 10 inch pie plate. Carefully remove the parchment paper.

3. Bake for around 15 minutes or until the edges are slightly brown. Remove from oven and allow crust to come to room temperature before filling.

4. Can be made 1-2 days in advance. Cover tightly and store in refrigerator.

Sexy Chocolate Cake

Total Time: 1hr 10 min
Prep: 10 min
Cook: 1hr

6 Servings
1 Whole-Food Fat Per Serving
1 Other Fats

Ingredients

- 1/2 cup SANE Cocoa Powder
- 1/2 cup coconut flour
- 2 1/2 teaspoons baking powder
- 1/2 teaspoon ground cinnamon Pinch of sea salt

- 6 eggs
- 1/2 cup SANE honey
- 1/2 cup extra virgin coconut oil
- 1/2 cup coconut milk
- 1 teaspoon vanilla paste

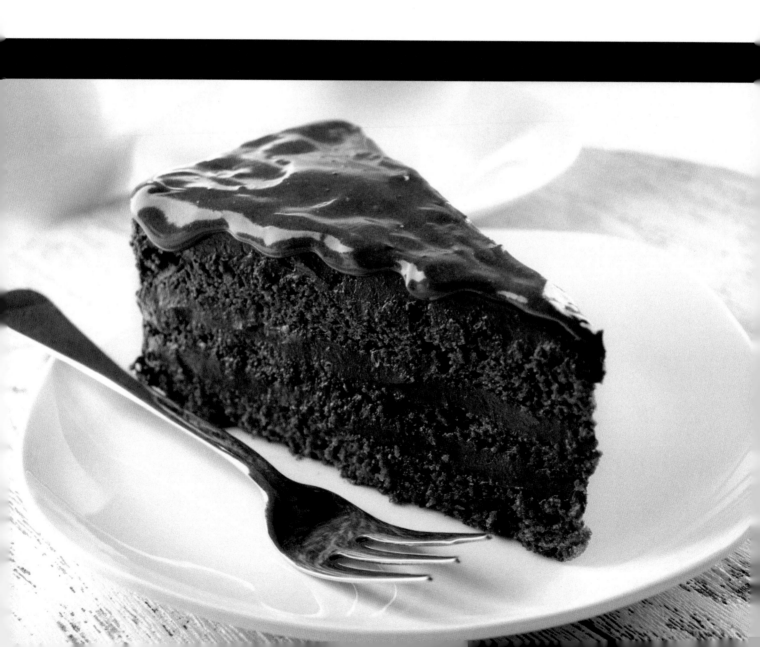

Directions

1. Preheat oven to 160°C (320°F)

2. Combine the SANE Cocoa Powder, coconut flour, baking powder, cinnamon and sea salt into a mixing bowl.

3. Add the eggs, SANE honey, vanilla, coconut milk and extra virgin coconut oil.

4. Mix well until smooth and combined – a whisk works well for this.

5. Pour into a 20 cm (9 inch) baking tin lined with baking paper.

6. Bake the cake for 55 – 60 minutes or until cooked through.

7. Best to test after 45 to make sure as oven temps may vary.

8. Remove from the oven and cool.

9. Spread with ganache or healthy chocolate mousse and enjoy.

SHORTBREAD COOKIES

Total Time: 15 min
Prep: 5 min
Cook: 10 min

6 Servings
1 Whole-Food Fat Per Serving

Ingredients

- 6 tbs coconut flour
- 4 tbs extra virgin coconut oil, melted

- 1-2 tbs SANE honey
- 1/4 tsp almond extract

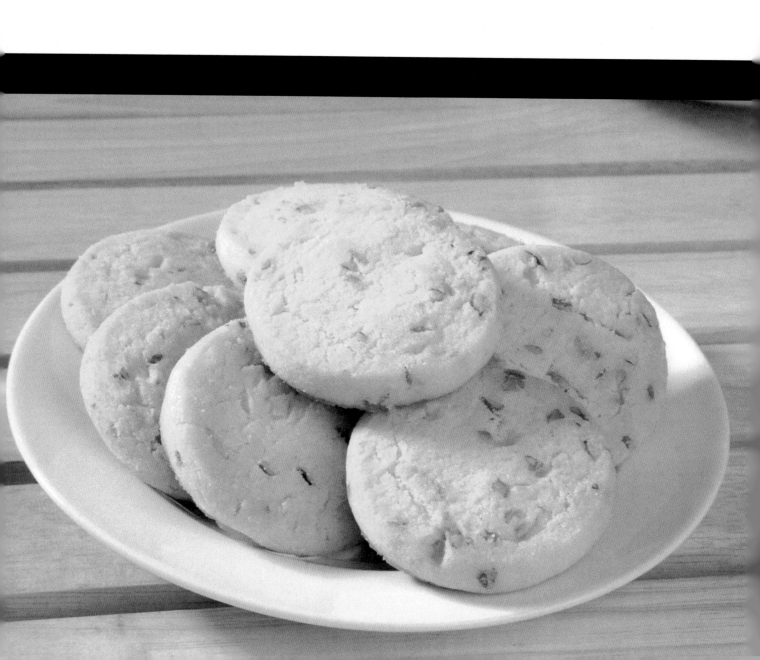

Directions

1. Preheat oven to 350 degrees.

2. In a small bowl, mix all ingredients together until it is the consistency of a thick paste.

3. Shape into balls and place on a lined baking sheet. press down on the tops gently with a fork.

4. Bake for 8-10 minutes until lightly browned on the bottom.

5. Let cool completely on the pan or they will crumble.

SNICKERDOODLE CUPCAKES

Total Time: 47 min
Prep: 25 min
Cook: 22 min

8 Servings
2 Whole-Food Fats Per Serving

Ingredients

- 3/4 cup Unsalted Butter
- 1 cup Xylitol
- 2 large Eggs (Whole)
- 2 tsps Vanilla Extract
- 3 tbsps Coconut cream

- 1 fl oz Tap Water
- 1 cup Almond Flour
- 3/4 tsp Baking Powder
- 1/8 tsp Salt
- 2 tsps Cinnamon
- 2 large Egg Whites

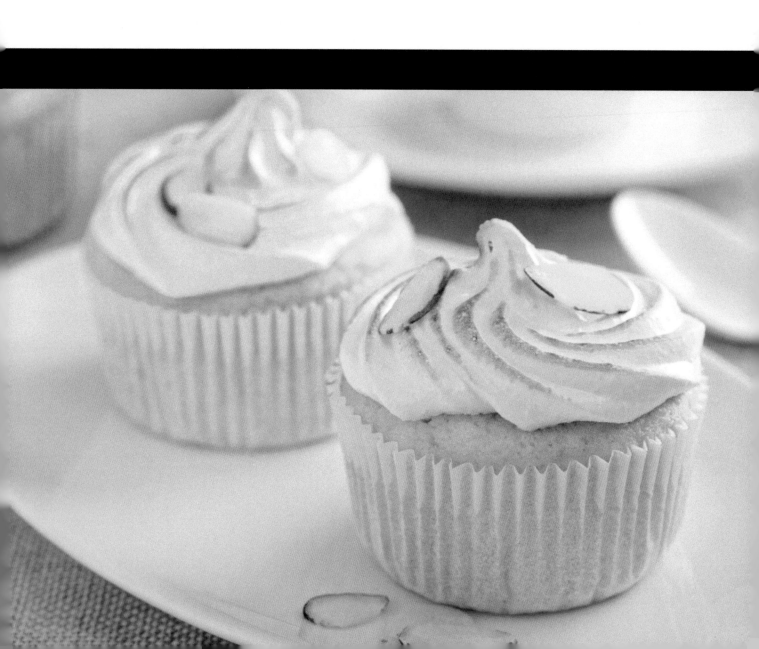

Directions

Cupcakes:

1. Preheat oven to 350°F. Prepare a muffin tin with 8 foil or paper liners. Beat 1/4 cup softened butter and 1/4 cup xylitol until light and fluffy.

2. Add 2 whole eggs, 1 tsp vanilla, coconut cream, 2 Tbsp water and almond flour.

3. In a separate bowl whisk to combine the 4 tbsps almond flour, baking powder, salt and 2 tsp cinnamon.

4. Combine the almond mixture with the egg mixture and blend until smooth.

5. Fill the muffin wells and bake for 20-25 minutes until cooked through.

6. Allow to sit in the muffin tin for 5 minutes then remove to a baking rack to cool. Frost once cooled.

Buttercream Frosting:

1. Prepare a pan with simmering water fitted with another pan over the top (Bain Marie).

2. Do not allow the surface of the water to touch the bottom of the top pan.

3. To the top pan (a metal mixing bowl works great for this purpose) add 2 egg whites (be sure there are no yolks), a dash of coconut cream, 1 tsp water and the remaining of xylitol.

4. Whisk this mixture continuously for 5-10 minutes over the water bath until all the xylitol has dissolved.

5. Pour this mixture into a separate bowl and whip with a blender until stiff fluffy peaks form.

6. Add 1 tsp vanilla, blend to incorporate. The frosting may be used, as is, immediately (it does not store well) as a marshmallow frosting – dust the cupcakes with cinnamon as a garnish.

7. For butter cream: to the marshmallow frosting, continue to beat on medium speed, begin adding about 1/2 cup butter 1 tablespoon at a time (allow to beat for 1 minute in-between each addition of butter).

8. The frosting may break down and get soupy looking, continue to add butter and beat until it comes together (more butter may be necessary, 1 tablespoon at a time).

9. Add 1-2 tsp cinnamon (to taste, optional) and blend to combine.

10. Buttercream should be used immediately by piping onto the cooled cupcake with a pastry bag and fancy tip or by simply cutting the corner of a plastic bag.

11. Buttercream frosted cupcakes may be refrigerated in an airtight container for up to 5 days.

12. Serve at room temperature dusted with cinnamon.

Improve Your Weight Loss, Energy, Mood, and Digestion In Just 17 Second A Day!

 0g Sugar

 100% Plant-Based

 Gluten Free

 No GMO's

 No Dairy

 No Soy

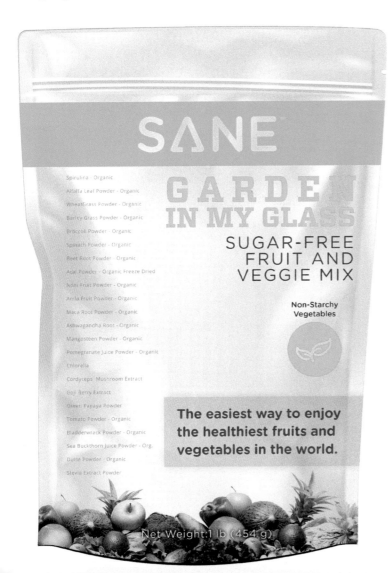

Introducing *Garden In My Glass*. The quickest, easiest, and most affordable way to get your family eating their fruits and veggies...and loving it!

When you order today you will also receive our wildly popular *'28 Days Of Green Smoothies'* recipe collection.

Plus, Get A Green Smoothie Recipe Book for FREE!

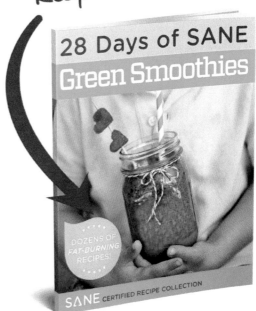

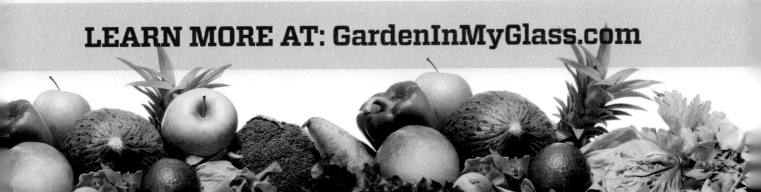

STRAWBERRIES CREAM CUPCAKES

Total Time: 30 min
Prep: 10 min
Cook: 20 min

10 Servings
3 Whole-Food Fats Per Serving

Ingredients

- 7 ozs Unsalted Butter
- 3/4 cup Xylitol
- 3 large Eggs (Whole)
- 1 tsp Vanilla Extract
- 1 1/4 Coconut Cream
- 1 1/2 fl ozs Tap Water

- 1 1/3 cup Almond Flour
- 1 tsp Baking Powder
- 1/4 tsp Salt
- 2 tbsps Sugar Free Strawberry Jam
- 10 small Strawberries

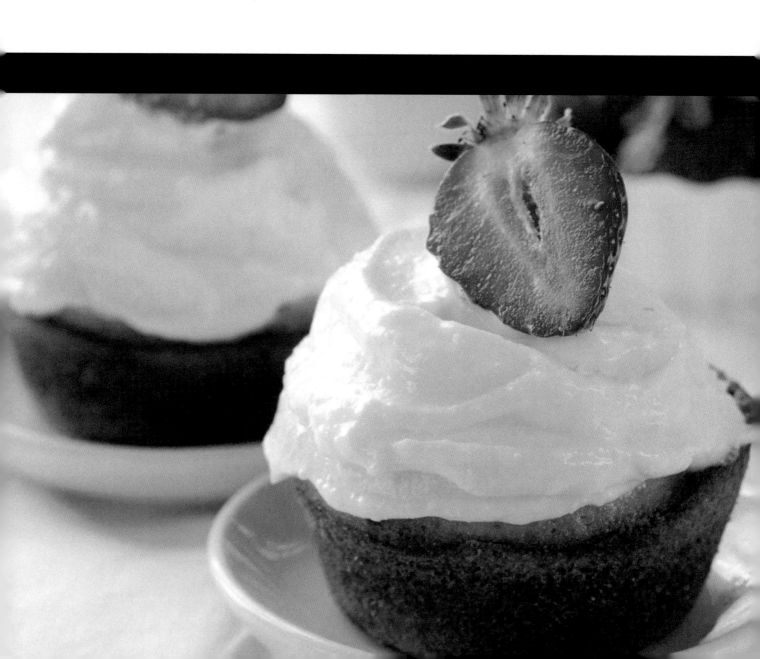

Directions

1. Preheat oven to 350°F. Line a muffin tin with 10 paper or foil liners. Beat 1/3 cup (about 3 oz) softened butter and xylitol until light and fluffy, about 3 minutes.

2. Add one egg at a time until incorporated, then the vanilla.

3. Add the almond flour and blend until incorporated. Add the coconut cream and water and continue to blend until smooth.

4. Combine the almond flour, baking powder and 1/4 tsp salt. Add to the egg mixture forming a thickened batter.

5. Divide equally into the 10 muffin liners and bake for 20-25 minutes until golden brown on top and baked through. Allow to cool.

Frosting:

1. Beat 1/2 cup (about 4 oz) butter, coconut cream and a dash of salt for about 2 minutes. Add 1/2 cup xylitol and 2 tablespoons sugar-free strawberry jam. 2-3 drops of red food coloring may be added for a pinker color.

2. Using a piping bag and fancy tip or simply a quart-sized plastic bag with a corner cut off, pipe the frosting onto the cupcakes and garnish with a strawberry.

3. The cupcakes can be kept in an airtight container refrigerated for up to one week. Serve at room temperature.

STRAWBERRY GRANITA

Total Time: 2hr
Prep: 2hr
Cook: 0 min

6 Servings
1 Low-Fructose Fruits Per Serving

Ingredients

- 16 ozs Strawberries
- 1 cup Tap Water
- 3/4 cup Xylitol
- 1 tbsp Fresh Lemon Juice

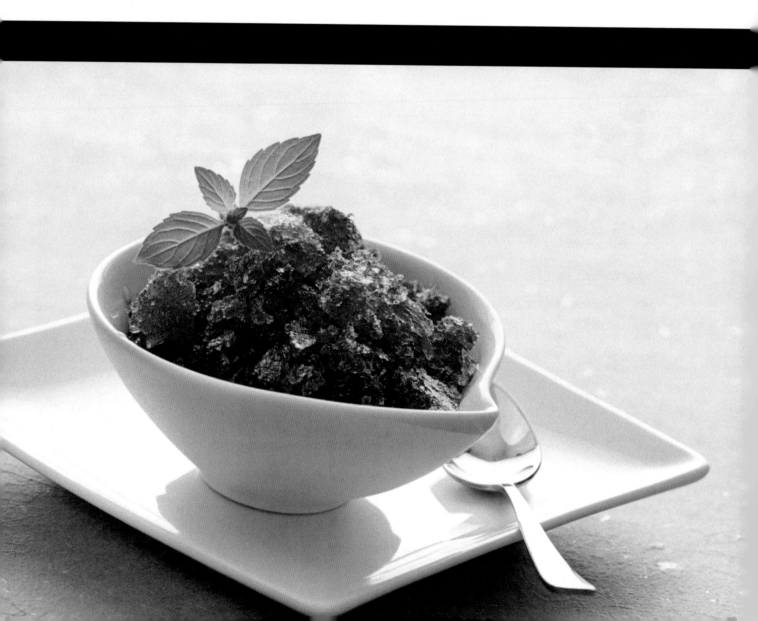

Directions

1. In a food processor fitted with a steel blade, purée the strawberries. Add water, xylitol and lemon juice. Pulse to combine.

2. Pour mixture into a 9 by 13-inch baking pan. Place in freezer. Freeze 30 minutes.

3. Stir with fork. Freeze an additional 1 ½ to 2 hours, scraping with a fork every 30 minutes (mixture should be granular) and breaking up any large pieces.

4. Serve in dessert bowls and garnish with mint sprigs, if desired.

STRAWBERRY SHORTCAKE TRIFLE

Total Time: 2hr
Prep: 1hr 40 min
Cook: 20 min

12 Servings
3 Whole-Food Fats Per Serving

Ingredients

- 1 1/2 cups Almond Flour
- 1 tsp Baking Powder
- 3 cups Coconut Cream
- 4 tbsps Xylitol
- 2 large Eggs (Whole)

- 4 tsps Vanilla Extract
- 4 tbsps Sugar Free Apricot Preserves
- 2 cup sliceds Strawberries
- 1 oz Almonds
- 3 tbsps Unsalted Butter

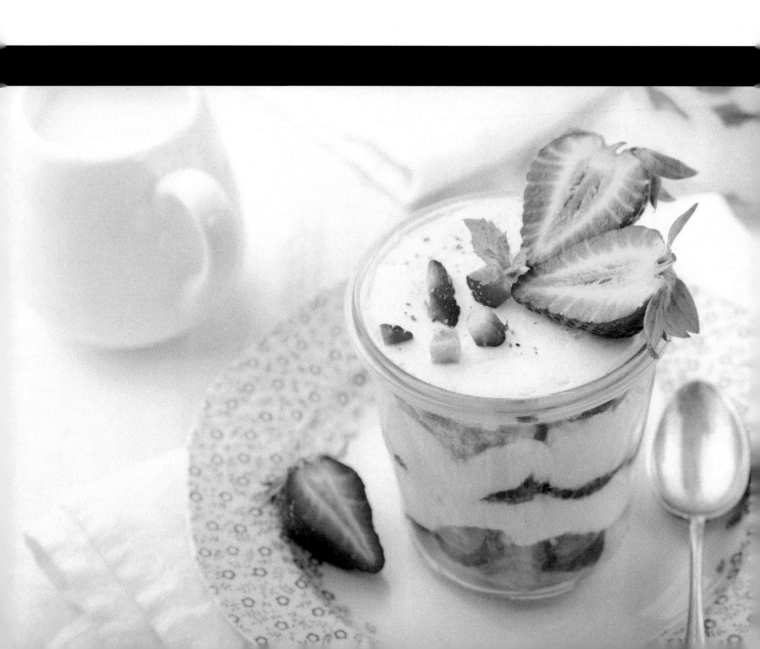

Directions

1. Preheat oven to 350°F. Spray a sheet pan with non-stick spray and set aside.

2. In a food processor, pulse the almond flour, baking powder and 2 teaspoons xylitol until mixed. Add the cold butter and pulse until it becomes crumbly. Add the eggs and 3 tablespoons of coconut cream and pulse until the mixture is thoroughly combined, about 30 seconds.

3. Drop about 2 tablespoons mixture onto the sheet pan making 12 rounded biscuits. Bake for 20 minutes until tops crack and are golden on the edges. Allow to cool.

4. In a medium bowl beat the remaining cream, 2 tablespoons xylitol and 2 teaspoons vanilla extract until soft peaks form, about 3 to 4 minutes. Place one-third of the coconut cream in a small bowl and set aside.

5. Whisk 2 tablespoons xylitol and 2 teaspoons vanilla extract into coconut cream. With a rubber spatula, gently fold cream cheese into the remaining two-thirds of the coconut cream until well combined. Set aside. Cut biscuits in half. Spread each with about 1 teaspoon jam, then cut into 1-inch pieces.

To assemble:

1. Spread one-third of the biscuit pieces on the bottom of a 2-quart glass dessert dish.

2. Spread half of the coconut cream mixture over biscuit pieces and top with 1 cup strawberries. Repeat.

3. Scatter remaining biscuit pieces over last layer of berries. Cover with reserved coconut cream. Top with remaining berries and scatter the toasted almonds on top. Chill for 1 hour for flavors to blend.

STRAWBERRY-RHUBARB PIE

Total Time: 2hr 40 min
Prep: 2hr 25 min
Cook: 15 min

8 Servings
1 Whole-Food Fat Per Serving

Ingredients

- 4 stalks Rhubarb
- 1/2 cup Tap Water
- 1/3 cup Xylitol
- 3 1/2 cup halves Strawberries
- 1/2 tsp Guar Gum
- 1/2 tsp Fresh Lemon Juice
- 1/8 tsp Salt
- 8 serving SANE Pie Crust

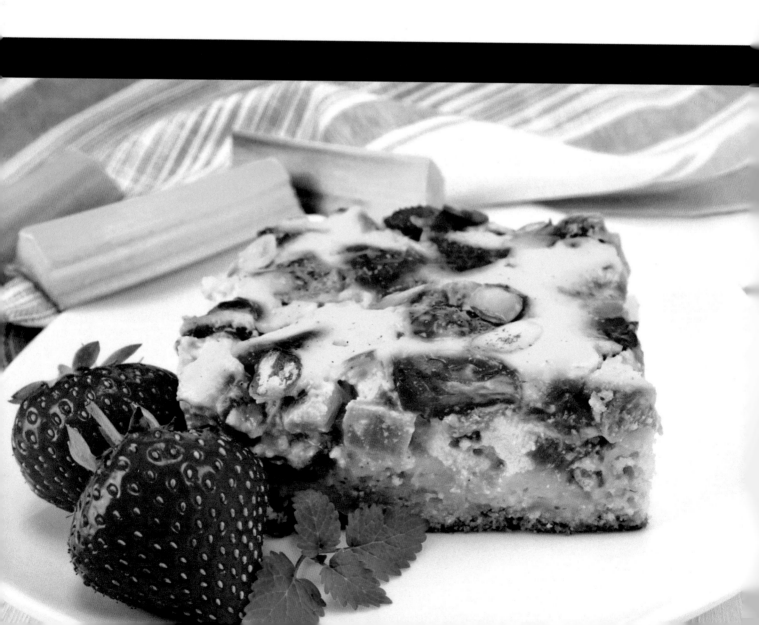

Directions

1. Prepare SANE Pie Crust according to recipe. Pre-bake the pie shell.

2. Chop rhubarb into 1-inch pieces and place it in a medium saucepan over medium heat with the water and xylitol. Bring to a boil. Reduce the heat and simmer until rhubarb is very soft, about 10 to 15 minutes. Turn heat down to low.

3. Add berries, thickener, lemon juice and salt and stir until thickened, about 3 minutes. Pour filling into prepared pie shell.

4. Chill until set, about 2 hours. Serve with coconut cream, if desired. Makes 8 servings.

Super Chocolate Chip Cookies

Total Time: 30 min
Prep: 20 min
Cook: 10 min

36 Servings
1 Whole-Food Fat Per Serving

Ingredients

- 1 tsp Baking Powder
- 1/2 tsp Salt
- 1 cup Salted Butter
- 1 cup Xylitol

- 2 tsps Vanilla Extract
- 2 large Eggs (Whole)
- 2 cups All Purpose SANE Baking Mix
- 6 ozs SANE Chocolate Chips

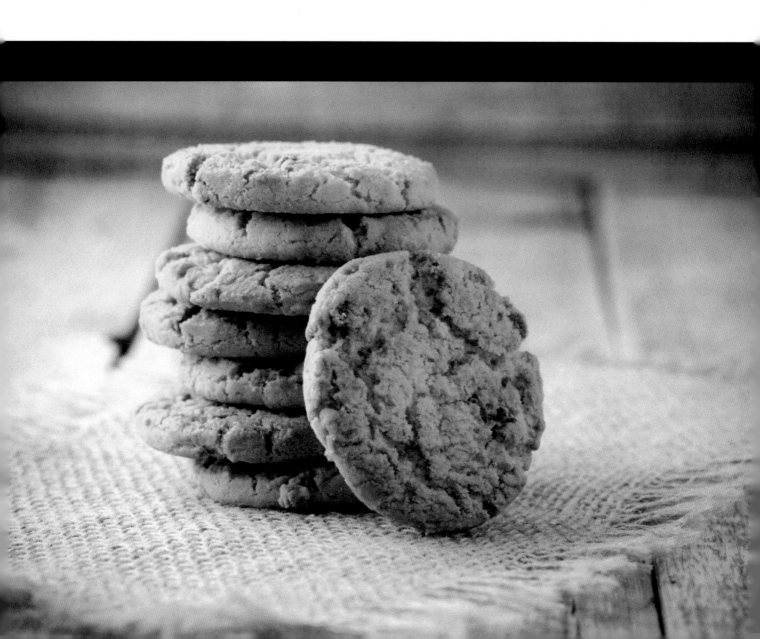

Directions

1. Preheat oven to 375°F.

2. Blend all dry ingredients together in a small mixing bowl, set aside.

3. Mix melted butter, xylitol and vanilla at medium speed with an electric mixer until well blended. Add eggs one at a time, mixing well after each addition. Gradually add dry ingredient mixture, beating until blended. Gently mix in chocolate chips with a wooden spoon or spatula.

4. Spoon rounded teaspoonfuls of cookie dough onto a cookie sheet coated with non-stick vegetable oil spray. Gently flatten cookies by pressing with hand or spatula.

5. Cook at 375° F for 10 to 12 minutes or until done or until lightly browned. Remove from baking sheet and place cookies on a wire rack to cool. (Do not overbake cookies or they will be dry and hard.)

TIRAMISU CUPCAKES

Total Time: 40 min
Prep: 25 min
Cook: 15 min

6 Servings
2 Whole-Food Fats Per Serving

Ingredients

- 3 tbsps Unsalted Butter
- 3 large Eggs (Whole)
- 9 tbsps Xylitol
- 4 tsps Vanilla Extract
- 1/4 cup Almond Flour
- 1/4 tsp Baking Powder
- 1/4 tsp Salt
- 4 ozs Mascarpone
- 1 1/4 tsp dries Coffee (Instant Powder)
- 1/2 cup Coconut Cream
- 1/2 fl oz Tap Water

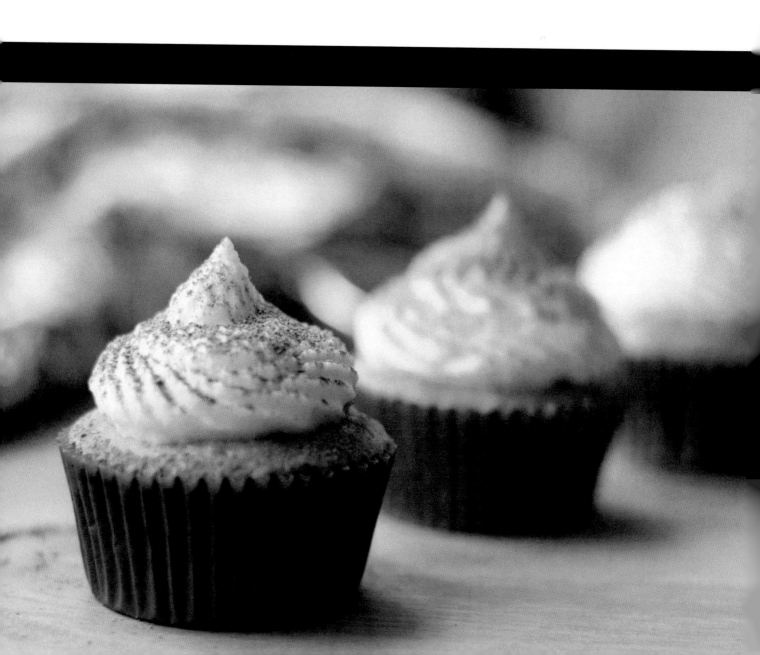

Directions

Cupcake

1. Preheat oven to 375°F. Prepare a muffin tin with paper or foil cups.

2. Using an electric mixer blend together the butter and 4 tbsps xylitol until light and fluffy; about 2 minutes. Add eggs, 1 tsp vanilla, almond flour, baking powder and salt. Blend until smooth then fill 6 muffin cups and bake for 15 minutes or until cooked through. Allow to sit for 5 minutes in the tin then place on a cooling rack.

3. Combine 2 tsp vanilla, 2 tbsps xylitol, 1 tsp espresso powder and 1 1/2 tbsps water.

4. Prick cupcakes with a tooth pick and pour 1 tsp soaking syrup per cupcake over the top.

Mascarpone Frosting

1. Beat together the mascarpone cheese, 3 tbsps xylitol, 1 tsp vanilla and 1/4 tsp espresso powder until smooth.

2. In a separate bowl whip the coconut cream until stiff peaks form.

3. Fold the coconut cream into the mascarpone mixture until combined. Place mixture in a pastry bag fitted with a fancy tip or simply use a plastic sandwich bag with a corner cut off. Pipe the frosting onto the cooled cupcakes.

4. Best if served the same day or they may be refrigerated overnight in an airtight container. Serve at room temperature dusted with SANE Cocoa Powder and topped with crushed espresso beans if desired.

VANILLA MOUSSE WITH RHUBARB

Total Time: 25 min
Prep: 15 min
Cook: 10 min

2 Servings
2 Whole-Food Fats Per Serving

Ingredients

- 2 stalks Rhubarb
- 1/4 cup Tap Water
- 1 tbsp Sugar Free Strawberry Jam

- 1/2 cup Coconut Cream
- 4 ozs Greek Yogurt - Plain (Container)
- 3 tsps Xylitol

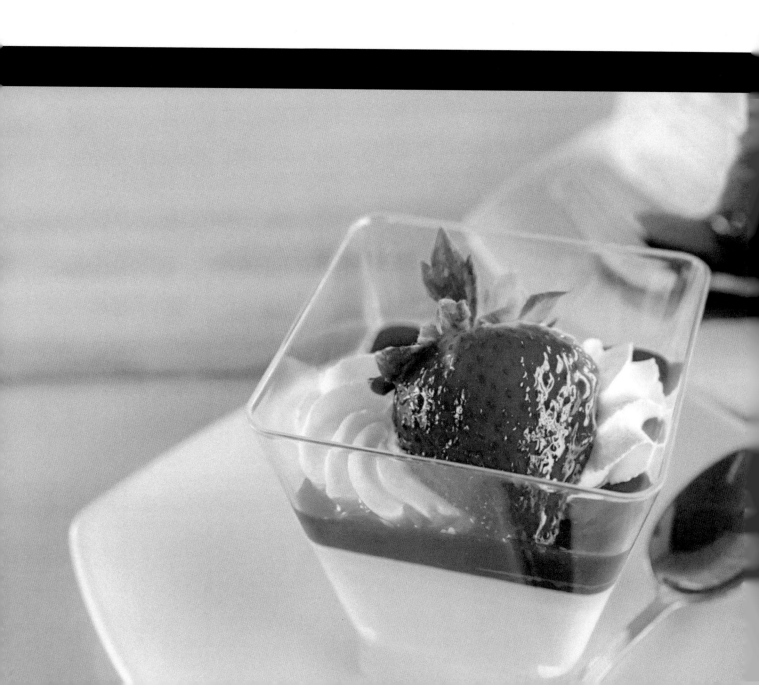

Directions

1. For the rhubarb sauce: In a small saucepan, combine the rhubarb, water and strawberry jam; bring to a simmer over medium heat. Reduce heat to medium-low; cover and simmer, stirring occasionally, until rhubarb is a sauce-like consistency, about 10 minutes. Set aside to cool.

2. For the vanilla mousse: In a mixing bowl, with an electric mixer on medium-high speed, beat together the coconut cream, 4 oz yogurt, and xylitol to semi-firm peaks. Reserve 1/4 cup mousse for topping.

3. To assemble: Set out two martini glasses or wineglasses. Spoon 1/4 cup mousse in the bottom of each glass and spread evenly. Top each with 1 1/2 tablespoons rhubarb sauce. Divide the remaining mousse between the glasses, then top with the remaining rhubarb. Top with the reserved 1/4 cup mousse, dividing evenly.

Walnut Blondies

Total Time: 50 min
Prep: 20 min
Cook: 30 min

12 Servings
2 Whole-Food Fats Per Serving

Ingredients

- 1 cup chopped English Walnuts
- 1 cup Unsalted Butter
- 1 cup Xylitol
- 1 tsp Vanilla Extract

- 1 1/2 Almond Flour
- 1 1/2 tsp Guar Gum
- 3 large Eggs (Whole)
- 1 1/2 tsps Baking Powder
- 1/2 tsp Cinnamon

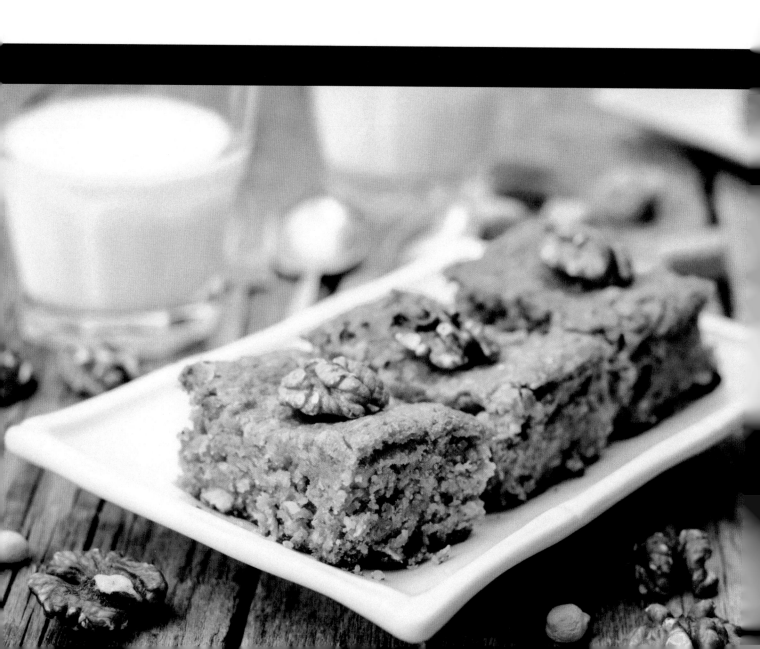

Directions

1. Heat oven to 325°F. Toast walnuts on a sheet pan for 8-10 minutes, cool and then coarsely chop. Set aside.

2. Line a 13-by-9-inch baking pan with aluminum foil extending 2 inches over both short sides of pan. Grease foil, and set aside.

3. Whisk butter, xylitol, eggs and vanilla extract together in a large bowl. In another bowl whisk almond flour, guar gum, baking powder and cinnamon together; stir into butter mixture until well combined. Stir in walnuts. Spread evenly into prepared pan. Bake until puffed and set, and a toothpick inserted in center comes out clean (top will not be browned), 30 minutes.

4. Cool completely in pan on a wire rack. Let stand until set, about 1 hour. (The recipe can be prepared up to this point, covered with plastic wrap and stored at room temperature overnight.)

5. Firmly gripping the foil on both ends, lift blondies out of pan, and place on work surface. Cut into 12 pieces, and serve.

WALNUT BROWNIES

Total Time: 40 min
Prep: 15 min
Cook: 25 min

16 Servings
1 Whole-Food Fat Per Serving

Ingredients

- 1/2 second spray coconut oil
- 1 cup Unsalted Butter
- 3 tbsps Xylitol
- 4 large Eggs (Whole)
- 1/2 cup Almond Flour
- 1/2 cup Tap Water
- 4 ozs Sugar Free Chocolate Chips
- 2 tsps Vanilla Extract
- 1 cup chopped English Walnuts

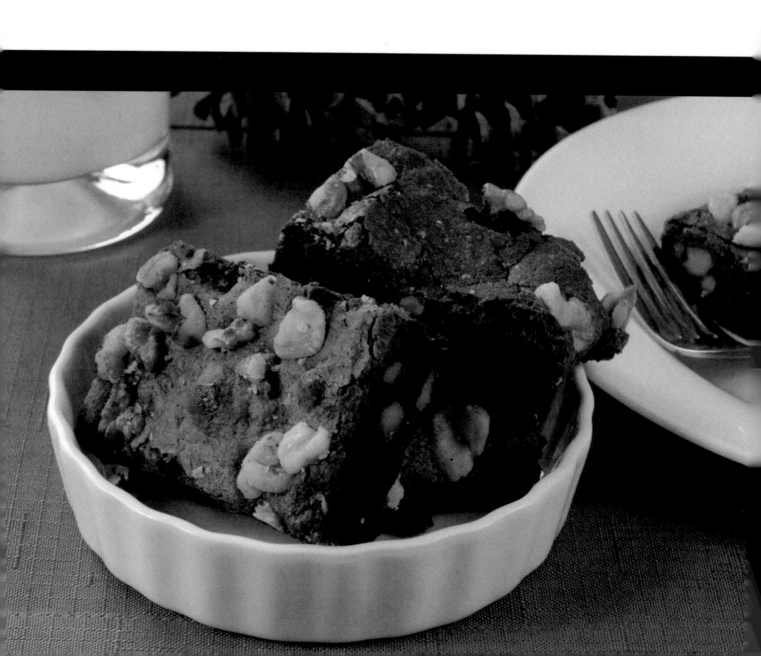

Directions

1. Preheat oven to 350°F. Line an 8 square baking pan with aluminum foil and spray with coconut cooking spray.

2. Melt chocolate over a double boiler or in the microwave and set aside to cool.

3. With an electric mixer on medium, beat butter and xylitol until light and creamy, about 4 minutes. Turn speed down to low and beat in eggs, one at a time. Add melted chocolate and blend well. Add almond flour, water, xylitol and extracts (3 tbsp chocolate extract is optional); mix until just combined. Fold in nuts. Transfer batter to prepared pan.

4. Bake 20 to 25 minutes, until a tester inserted in the center comes out with just a few crumbs. Cool and cut into 16 squares.

So Much To Look Forward To...

You will learn much more about this as we start your personal weight-loss plan together in your free half-day Masterclass (reserve your seat at SANESeminar.com), but here are a few key reminders as you're getting started on your SANE journey.

SANE eating is a lifelong, enjoyable, sustainable, simple, and delicious way of eating. **It is not a repackaging of the unsustainable calorie counting diets that failed you.**

I know you understand this already—otherwise you wouldn't be here—but please keep in mind that since SANE isn't a calorie counting diet, you will not suffer through the same calorie counting tools and resources that failed you in the past. For example, **memorizing endless food lists and following unrealistic minute-by-minute meal plans aren't just a pain— they cannot work in the real world**, and they cannot work long term.

Life is crazy. Things happen. And heck, people have different tastes in food, so while minute-by-minute "eat exactly this right now no matter what" endless lists might make for good reality TV, if they worked in the real world, you would have already met your goals. **To get a different result (long-term fat loss and robust health), you MUST take a different approach.** That's what you will find here.

If you approach your new SANE life calmly, gradually, and with the next 30 years in mind rather than the next 30 days, **you will learn the underlying principles that enable you to make the SANE choices easily—forever**.

Think of your new approach as the difference between memorizing the sum of every possible combination of numbers versus learning the underlying principles of how addition works. Once you understand addition, lists and memorization aren't necessary as you know what to do with any combination of numbers—forever.

The same thing applies with food. Once you understand the new science of SANE eating, **you will know exactly what to eat (and what to avoid) everywhere you go—forever—without any lists** or any memorization.

This new approach changes everything and will forever free you from all the confusing and conflicting weight-loss information you've been told. So please allow me to congratulate you on coming to the life-changing realization that **to get different results than you've gotten in the past, you must take a different approach than you used in the past!**

The great news is that when you combine a calm, gradual, long-term, and progress vs. perfection mindset with your scientifically proven SANE tools, program, and coaching, you are **guaranteed to burn belly fat, boost energy, and enjoy an unstoppable sense of self-confidence!**

Your new SANE lifestyle has helped over 100,000 people in over 37 countries burn fat and boost health *long-term*....and it will do the same for you if you let it and trust it.

Thank you for taking the road less travelled...it will make all the difference!

SANEly and Gratefully,

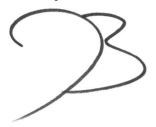

Jonathan Bailor | SANE Founder, NYTimes Bestselling Author, and soon...your personal weight-loss coach

P.S. Over the years I have found that our most successful members, the ones who have lost 60, 70, even 100 pounds... and kept it off... are the ones who start their personal weight-loss plan on...

our FREE half-day Masterclass. It's your best opportunity to fall in love with the SANE lifestyle, learn exactly how to start making the simple changes that lead to dramatic body transformations, and get introduced to your new SANE family. Be sure to reserve your spot at http://SANESeminar.com.

Please Don't Lose Your Seat at the FREE Masterclass Seminar!

Reserve your spot now so we can start your perfect personalized weight-loss plan. Space is limited and fills-up quickly. Reserve your spot now so you don't miss out!

Yes! I want to reserve my spot now at SANESeminar.com

About the Author: Jonathan Bailor is a New York Times bestselling author and internationally recognized natural weight loss expert who specializes in using modern science and technology to simplify health. Bailor has collaborated with top scientists for more than 10 years to analyze and apply over 1,300 studies. His work has been endorsed by top doctors and scientists from Harvard Medical School, Johns' Hopkins, The Mayo Clinic, The Cleveland Clinic, and UCLA.

Bailor is the founder of SANESolution.com and serves as the CEO for the wellness technology company Yopti®. He authored the New York Times and USA Today bestselling book *The Calorie Myth*, hosts a popular syndicated health radio show *The SANE Show*, and blogs on *The Huffington Post*. Additionally, Bailor has registered over 25 patents, spoken at Fortune 100 companies and TED conferences for over a decade, and served as a Senior Program Manager at Microsoft where he helped create Nike+ Kinect Training and XBox Fitness.

Made in the USA
Middletown, DE
12 May 2023